This report contains the collective views of an international group of experts and does not necessarily represent the decisions or the stated policy of the United Nations Environment Programme, the International Labour Organisation, or the World Health Organization.

Environmental Health Criteria 130

ENDRIN

First draft prepared by Dr G. T. van Esch, Bilthoven, Netherlands, and Dr E. A. H. van Heemstra-Lequin, Laren, Netherlands

Published under the joint sponsorship of the United Nations Environment Programme, the International Labour Organisation, and the World Health Organization

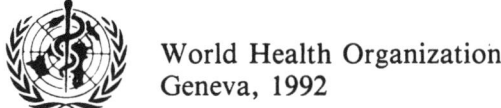

World Health Organization
Geneva, 1992

The **International Programme on Chemical Safety (IPCS)** is a joint venture of the United Nations Environment Programme, the International Labour Organisation, and the World Health Organization. The main objective of IPCS is to carry out and disseminate evaluations of the effects of chemicals on human health and the quality of the environment. Supporting activities include the development of epidemiological, experimental laboratory, and risk-assessment methods that could produce internationally comparable results, and the development of manpower in the field of toxicology. Other activities carried out by IPCS include the development of know-how for coping with chemical accidents, coordination of laboratory testing and epidemiological studies, and promotion of research on the mechanisms of the biological action of chemicals.

WHO Library Cataloguing in Publication Data
Endrin.
(Environmental health criteria ; 130)
1.Endrin—toxicity 2.Environmental exposure I.Series
ISBN 92 4 157130 6   (NLM Classification: WA 240)
ISSN 0250-863X

The World Health Organization welcomes requests for permission to reproduce or translate its publications, in part or in full. Applications and enquiries should be addressed to the Office of Publications, World Health Organization, Geneva, Switzerland, which will be glad to provide the latest information on any changes made to the text, plans for new editions, and reprints and translations already available.

© World Health Organization 1992

Publications of the World Health Organization enjoy copyright protection in accordance with the provisions of Protocol 2 of the Universal Copyright Convention. All rights reserved.

The designations employed and the presentation of the material in this publication do not imply the expression of any opinion whatsoever on the part of the Secretariat of the World Health Organization concerning the legal status of any country, territory, city, or area or of its authorities, or concerning the delimitation of its frontiers or boundaries.

The mention of specific companies or of certain manufacturers' products does not imply that they are endorsed or recommended by the World Health Organization in preference to others of a similar nature that are not mentioned. Errors and omissions excepted, the names of proprietary products are distinguished by initial capital letters.

CONTENTS

1. SUMMARY AND EVALUATION; CONCLUSIONS;
   RECOMMENDATIONS 13

   1.1 Summary and evaluation 13
       1.1.1 Exposure 13
       1.1.2 Uptake, metabolism, and excretion 14
       1.1.3 Effects on organisms in the environment 15
       1.1.4 Effects on experimental animals and *in vitro* ... 15
       1.1.5 Effects on human beings 17
   1.2 Conclusions 18
   1.3 Recommendations 18

2. IDENTITY, PHYSICAL AND CHEMICAL PROPERTIES,
   ANALYTICAL METHODS 20

   2.1 Identity 20
   2.2 Physical and chemical properties 21
   2.3 Conversion factors 22
   2.4 Analytical methods 22

3. SOURCES OF HUMAN AND ENVIRONMENTAL
   EXPOSURE 30

   3.1 Natural occurrence 30
   3.2 Man-made sources 30
       3.2.1 Production levels and processes, uses 30
             3.2.1.1 World production figures 30
             3.2.1.2 Manufacturing processes 31

4. ENVIRONMENTAL TRANSPORT, DISTRIBUTION, AND
   TRANSFORMATION 32

   4.1 Transport and distribution between media 32
       4.1.1 Air 32
       4.1.2 Water 32

				Page
		4.1.3	Soil	33
		4.1.4	Soil–plants	34
	4.2	Abiotic degradation		34
	4.3	Biotransformation		36
		4.3.1	Biodegradation	36
		4.3.2	Bioaccumulation and biomagnification	36

5. ENVIRONMENTAL LEVELS AND HUMAN EXPOSURE 41

    5.1 Environmental levels 41
        5.1.1 Air 41
        5.1.2 Soil, sediments, and sewage sludge 50
            5.1.2.1 Soil 50
            5.1.2.2 Sediments 50
            5.1.2.3 Sewage sludge 68
        5.1.3 Water 68
            5.1.3.1 Surface water 68
            5.1.3.2 Rain and snow 70
            5.1.3.3 Drinking-water 70
            5.1.3.4 Groundwater 71
        5.1.4 Organisms in the environement 71
            5.1.4.1 Birds 71
            5.1.4.2 Fish and shellfish 73
            5.1.4.3 Mixed species 75
        5.1.5 Other food and feed 76
            5.1.5.1 Cereals 76
            5.1.5.2 Fruit and vegetables 76
            5.1.5.3 Meat, poultry, and chicken eggs 77
            5.1.5.4 Milk and milk products 78
            5.1.5.5 Fat and oils 79
            5.1.5.6 Animal feed 80
        5.1.6 Miscellaneous products 80
    5.2 Exposure of the general population 80
        5.2.1 Total-diet studies 80
        5.2.2 Levels in human tissues 82
            5.2.2.1 Adipose tissue 82
            5.2.2.2 Organs 83
            5.2.2.3 Blood 83
            5.2.2.4 Breast milk 83
            5.2.2.5 Appraisal of exposure of the general population 84

	5.3	Occupational exposure during manufacture, formulation, and use	84
		5.3.1 Manufacture and formulation	84
		5.3.2 Application	85
		5.3.3 Appraisal of occupational exposure	87
6.	KINETICS AND METABOLISM		88
	6.1	Absorption, distribution, and elimination	88
		6.1.1 Laboratory animals	88
		6.1.1.1 Oral administration	88
		6.1.1.2 Intravenous administration	90
		6.1.2 Domestic animals	91
		6.1.3 Human beings	93
		6.1.4 Systems *in vitro*	93
	6.2	Biotransformation	93
		6.2.1 Experimental animals	93
		6.2.2 Human beings	96
		6.2.3 Microorganisms	97
		6.2.4 Plants	98
7.	EFFECTS ON ORGANISMS IN THE ENVIRONMENT		99
	7.1	Microorganisms	99
	7.2	Aquatic organisms	99
		7.2.1 Invertebrates	99
		7.2.2 Fish	106
		7.2.2.1 Acute toxicity	106
		7.2.2.2 Short-term toxicity	106
		7.2.2.3 Studies of resistance	114
		7.2.2.4 Interaction with other chemicals	115
		7.2.2.5 Special studies	116
		7.2.3 Amphibia	118
	7.3	Terrestrial organisms	118
		7.3.1 Honey bees	118
		7.3.2 Birds	119
		7.3.2.1 Acute toxicity	119
		7.3.2.2 Short-term toxicity	119
		7.3.2.3 Studies of reproduction	120
		7.3.2.4 Interaction with other chemicals	121
		7.3.2.5 Special studies	121
		7.3.2.6 Behavioural studies	122

	7.3.3	Mammals 122
		7.3.3.1 Toxicity 122
		7.3.3.2 Studies of resistance 123
	7.4	Effects in the field 124
	7.5	Appraisal of effects on organisms in the environment 126

8. EFFECTS ON EXPERIMENTAL ANIMALS AND *IN VITRO* 127

8.1	Acute toxicity of technical-grade endrin 127
	8.1.1 Oral administration 127
	8.1.2 Dermal administration 127
	8.1.3 Parenteral administration 127
	8.1.4 Toxicity of metabolites and isomers 131
	8.1.4.1 Mammalian metabolites 131
	8.1.4.2 Isomers 132
	8.1.5 Acute toxicity of formulated material 133
	8.1.5.1 Oral and dermal administration 133
	8.1.5.2 Inhalation 133
8.2	Short-term exposure 134
	8.2.1 Oral administration 134
	8.2.1.1 Mouse 134
	8.2.1.2 Rat 134
	8.2.1.3 Rabbit 135
	8.2.1.4 Dog 135
	8.2.1.5 Domestic animals 136
	8.2.2 Inhalation 137
	8.2.3 Dermal administration 137
8.3	Skin irritation 137
8.4	Reproduction, embryotoxicity, and teratogenicity 137
	8.4.1 Reproduction 137
	8.4.1.1 Mouse 137
	8.4.1.2 Rat 138
	8.4.2 Embryotoxicity and teratogenicity 138
	8.4.2.1 Mouse 138
	8.4.2.2 Rat 139
	8.4.2.3 Hamster 140
	8.4.2.4 Perinatal behavioural development ... 141
	8.4.3 Appraisal of reproductive effects 142
8.5	Mutagenicity and related end-points 142
	8.5.1 Effects on microorganisms 142
	8.5.2 Point mutations in mammalian cells 144

	8.5.3	Dominant lethal mutations 144
	8.5.4	Chromosomal and cytogenetic effects 144
	8.5.5	Host-mediated effects 145
	8.5.6	Sister chromatid exchange 145
	8.5.7	Effects in *Drosophila melanogaster* 145
	8.5.8	Effects on DNA 146
	8.5.9	Appraisal of mutagenicity and related end-points 146
8.6	Long-term exposure 147
8.7	Carcinogenicity 147
	8.7.1	Oral administration 147
		8.7.1.1 Mouse 147
		8.7.1.2 Rat 148
		8.7.1.3 Tumour promotion 150
	8.7.2	Appraisal of carcinogenicity 150
8.8	Special studies 151
	8.8.1	Nervous system 151
		8.8.1.1 Electrophysiological studies 151
		8.8.1.2 Histopathological studies 152
		8.8.1.3 Neurotransmitter systems 152
		8.8.1.4 Appraisal of effects on the nervous system 155
	8.8.2	Cardiovascular system 155
	8.8.3	Effects on liver enzymes 156
		8.8.3.1 Mouse 156
		8.8.3.2 Rat 157
		8.8.3.3 Guinea-pig 158
		8.8.3.4 In-vitro studies 158
	8.8.4	Miscellaneous studies 159
	8.8.5	Factors that influence toxicity 159
		8.8.5.1 Nutrition 159
		8.8.5.2 Potentiation 160

9. **EFFECTS ON HUMAN BEINGS** 162

    9.1 Exposure of the general population 162
         9.1.1 Acute toxicity 162
         9.1.2 Poisoning incidents 162
    9.2 Occupational exposure 165
         9.2.1 Factory workers 165
         9.2.2 Dose–response relationships 167
         9.2.3 Exposures to mixtures 168
         9.2.4 Appraisal of effects of occupational exposures 170

10. PREVIOUS EVALUATIONS BY INTERNATIONAL BODIES ... 171

REFERENCES 173

ANNEX I   Chemical names of endrin and its metabolites 218
ANNEX II   Medical treatment of endrin poisoning................................. 221
ANNEX III Management of major status epilepticus in adults 223

RESUME 226
RESUMEN 234

WHO TASK GROUP ON ENVIRONMENTAL HEALTH CRITERIA FOR ENDRIN

Members

Dr L.A. Albert, Consultores Ambientales Asociados, Xalapa, Veracruz, Mexico

Dr V. Benes, Department of Toxicology and Reference Laboratory, Institute of Hygiene and Epidemiology, Prague, Czechoslovakia

Dr S. Dobson, Institute of Terrestrial Ecology, Monks Wood Experimental Station, Huntingdon, United Kingdom

Dr G.J. van Esch, Bilthoven, Netherlands (*Rapporteur*)

Dr E.A.H. van Heemstra-Lequin, Laren, Netherlands (*Rapporteur*)

Dr S.K. Kashyap, National Institute of Occupational Health, Ahmedabad, India

Dr Yu.I. Kundiev, Research Institute of Labour Hygiene and Occupational Diseases, Kiev, Ukraine (*Vice-Chairman*)

Dr Y. Osman, Ministry of Health, Riyadh, Saudi Arabia

Dr H. Spencer, United States Environmental Protection Agency, Washington DC, USA (*Chairman*)

Dr C. Winder, National Institute of Occupational Health and Safety, Forest Lodge, New South Wales, Australia

Secretariat

Dr K.W. Jager, International Programme on Chemical Safety, World Health Organization, Geneva, Switzerland (*Secretary*)

Ms B. Labarthe, International Register of Potentially Toxic Chemicals, United Nations Environment Programme, Geneva, Switzerland

Dr T.K. Ng, Office of Occupational Health, World Health Organization, Geneva, Switzerland

NOTE TO READERS OF THE CRITERIA MONOGRAPHS

Every effort has been made to present information in the Criteria monographs as accurately as possible without unduly delaying their publication. In the interest of all users of the Environmental Health Criteria monographs, readers are kindly requested to communicate any errors that may have occurred to the Director of the International Programme on Chemical Safety, World Health Organization, Geneva, Switzerland, in order that they may be included in corrigenda.

* * *

A detailed data profile and a legal file can be obtained from the International Register of Potentially Toxic Chemicals, Palais des Nations, 1211 Geneva 10, Switzerland (Telephone no. 7988400 or 7985850).

* * *

The proprietary information contained in this monograph cannot replace documentation for registration purposes, because the latter has to be closely linked to the source, the manufacturing route, and the purity/impurities of the substance to be registered. The data should be used in accordance with paragraphs 82–84 and recommendations paragraph 90 of the Second FAO Government Consultation (1982).

ENVIRONMENTAL HEALTH CRITERIA FOR ENDRIN

A WHO Task Group on Environmental Health Criteria for Endrin and Isobenzan met at the World Health Organization, Geneva, from 23 to 27 July 1990. Dr K.W. Jager, IPCS, welcomed the participants on behalf of Dr M. Mercier, Director of IPCS, and the three IPCS cooperating organizations (UNEP, ILO, WHO). The Group reviewed and revised the draft Criteria monographs and Health and Safety Guides and made an evaluation of the risks to human health and the environment from exposure to endrin and isobenzan.

The first drafts of these monographs were prepared in cooperation between Dr E.A.H. van Heemstra-Lequin and Dr G.J. van Esch of the Netherlands. Dr van Esch prepared the second drafts, incorporating the comments received following circulation of the first drafts to the IPCS contact points for Environmental Health Criteria monographs.

Dr K.W. Jager of the IPCS Central Unit was responsible for the scientific content of the monographs, and Mrs E. Heseltine, St Léon-sur-Vézère, France, for the editing.

The fact that Shell Oil Co. made available to IPCS and the Task Group proprietary toxicological information on their products is gratefully acknowledged. This allowed the Task Group to base their evaluation on more complete data.

The effort of all who helped in the preparation and finalization of the monographs is gratefully acknowledged.

* * *

Partial financial support for the publication of this Criteria monograph was kindly provided by the United States Department of Health and Human Services, through a contract from the National Institute of Environmental Health Sciences, Research Triangle Park, North Carolina, USA, a WHO Collaborating Centre for Environmental Health Effects.

1. SUMMARY AND EVALUATION; CONCLUSIONS; RECOMMENDATIONS

1.1 Summary and evaluation

1.1.1 Exposure

Endrin is an organochlorine insecticide which has been used since the 1950s against a wide range of agricultural pests, mostly on cotton but also on rice, sugar-cane, maize, and other crops. It is also used as a rodenticide. It is available commercially as dusts, granules, pastes, and an emulsifiable concentrate.

Endrin enters the air mainly by volatilization and aerial drift. In general, volatilization takes place after application to soils and crops and depends on many factors, such as the organic matter and moisture content of the soil, humidity, air flow, and the surface area of plants.

The most important route of contamination of surface water is run-off from soil. Contamination from precipitation in the form of snow or rain is negligible. Local contamination of the environment may occur from industrial effluents and careless application practices.

The major source of endrin in soil is from direct application to soil and crops. Endrin can be retained, transported, or degraded in soil, depending on a number of factors. The greatest retention occurs in soils with a high content of organic matter. The persistence of endrin is highly dependent upon local conditions; its half-life in soil can range up to 12 years. Volatilization and photodecomposition are the primary factors in the disappearance of endrin from soil surfaces. Under the influence of sunlight (ultraviolet light), the isomer delta-ketoendrin is formed. In intense summer sun, about 50% of endrin was isomerized to this ketoendrin within 7 days. Microbial transformation (in fungi and bacteria) takes place, especially under anaerobic conditions, to give the same product.

Aquatic invertebrates and fish take up endrin rapidly from water, but exposed fish transferred to uncontaminated water lose the pesticide rapidly. Bioconcentration factors of 14–18 000 have been recorded after continuous exposure. Soil invertebrates may also take up endrin readily.

Summary and evaluation; conclusions; recommendations

The occasional presence of low levels of endrin in air and in surface and drinking-water in agricultural areas is of little significance from the point of view of public health. The only exposure that may be relevant is dietary intake. In general, however, the reported intake levels are far below the acceptable daily intake of 0.0002 mg/kg body weight established in 1970 (FAO/WHO, 1971).

1.1.2 Uptake, metabolism, and excretion

Unlike dieldrin, its stereoisomer, endrin is metabolized rapidly by animals, and very little is accumulated in fat in comparison with compounds of similar chemical structure.

Both uptake and excretion after oral administration are rapid in rats, and its biological half-life is 1–6 days, depending on the dose level. A steady state, at which the excreted amount equals the daily intake, is reached after 6 days. A sex difference is observed, in that males excrete endrin and metabolites via the bile much faster than females, resulting in less accumulation in male adipose tissue. Rats excrete this compound mainly in the faeces as endrin, *anti*-12-hydroxyendrin, and a hydroxylated endrin derivative within the first 24 h (70–75%); a third metabolite, 12-ketoendrin, accumulates in tissues. Rabbits excrete 50% of the metabolites of endrin in urine, whereas in rats only 2% are excreted by this route; only unchanged endrin is found in the faeces of rabbits.

Cows administered endrin at 0.1 mg/kg of diet for 21 days excreted up to 65% as metabolites in urine, 20% in faeces, partly as unchanged endrin, and 3% in milk, also mainly as endrin. These cows had residue levels of 0.003–0.006 mg/litre in milk, 0.001–0.002 mg/kg in meat, and 0.02–0.1 mg/kg in fat.

Laying hens fed endrin showed residue levels (depending on the doses given) of up to 0.1 mg/kg in meat, 1 mg/kg in fat, 0.1–0.2 mg/kg in eggs (yolk), 0.4 mg/kg in kidney, and 0.5 mg/kg in liver. Except in liver and kidney, the residues found were mainly unchanged endrin. About 50% of the administered endrin was excreted in faeces, mainly as metabolites.

In human beings, rats, rabbits, cows, and hens, the major biotransformed metabolite of endrin is *anti*-12-hydroxyendrin, together with its sulfate and glucuronide conjugates. Four other metabolites were found but in only minor quantities. Mainly unchanged endrin is found in body tissues and milk. After this pesticide was applied to plants, unchanged endrin and two hydrophilic transformation products were identified.

1.1.3 Effects on organisms in the environment

The effect of endrin on soil bacteria and fungi is minimal. Dose levels of 10–1000 mg/kg of soil had no effect on decomposition of organic matter, denitrification, or generation of methane. Endrin is very toxic to fish, aquatic invertebrates, and phytoplankton: the 96-h LC_{50} values are mostly below 1.0 µg/litre. The lowest observed adverse effect level in a life cycle test on the mysid shrimp, *Mysidopsis bahia*, was established at 30 ng/litre.

The reported tests on the acute toxicity of endrin in aquatic organisms were conducted in aquaria without sediment; the presence of sediment would be expected to attenuate the effect of endrin. Heavily contaminated sediment had little effect on species living in open water, suggesting that sediment-bound endrin has low bioavailability. Tests have not been conducted on aquatic animals living in sediment.

The LD_{50} for terrestrial mammals and birds is in the order of 1.0–10.0 mg/kg body weight. Mallard ducks fed up to 3.0 mg/kg body weight for 12 weeks showed no effect on egg production, fertility, or hatchability.

Certain species of aquatic invertebrates, fish, and small mammals have been reported to be resistant to the toxicity of endrin, and exposure to several different organochlorine pesticides led to selection of strains resistant to endrin.

Fish kills were observed in areas of agricultural run-off and industrial discharge; and declining populations of brown pelicans (in Louisiana, USA) and of sandwich terns (in the Netherlands) have been attributed to exposure to endrin in combination with other halogenated chemicals.

1.1.4 Effects on experimental animals and in vitro

Endrin is a highly toxic pesticide, the signs of intoxication being neurotoxic. The oral LD_{50} of technical-grade endrin for laboratory animals is in the range of 3–43 mg/kg body weight; the dermal LD_{50} for rats is 5–20 mg/kg body weight. No substantial difference in acute oral or dermal toxicity was found between technical-grade and formulated (emulsifiable concentrate and wettable powder) products.

Summary and evaluation; conclusions; recommendations

Short-term experiments for oral toxicity have been carried out using mice, rats, rabbits, dogs, and domestic animals. In mice and rats, the maximum tolerated doses for 6 weeks were 5 and 15 mg/kg diet (equivalent to 0.7 mg/kg body weight), respectively. Rats survived a 16-week exposure to 1 mg/kg diet (equivalent to 0.05 mg/kg body weight); rabbits died after receiving repeated doses of 1 mg/kg body weight. In dogs, a dose of 1 mg/kg of diet (approximately equivalent to 0.025 mg/kg body weight), given over 2 years, was without effect.

The neurological basis of the observed signs of intoxication is inhibition of gamma-aminobutyric acid (GABA) function at low doses. Like other chlorinated hydrocarbon insecticides, endrin also affects the liver, and stimulation of enzyme systems involved in the metabolism of other chemicals is evident, as shown by, for instance, decreased hexobarbital sleeping time in mice.

Doses of 75–150 mg/kg applied dermally as a dry powder for 2 h daily caused convulsions and death in rabbits but did not result in skin irritation. Production of systemic toxicity without irritation at the site of contact is noteworthy.

Long-term studies of toxicity and carcinogenicity have been performed in mice and rats. No carcinogenic effect was found, but these studies had shortcomings, including poor survival of the animals. The no-observed-effect level for toxicity in a two-year study in rats was 1 mg/kg of diet (equivalent to about 0.05 mg/kg body weight). Tumour promoting effects were not demonstrated when endrin was tested in combination with subminimal quantities of chemicals known to be carcinogenic to animals. The Task Group concluded that the data are insufficient to indicate that endrin is a carcinogenic hazard to humans.

Endrin was found to be nonmutagenic in several studies.

In most studies, it was not teratogenic to mice, rats, or hamsters, even at doses that caused maternal or fetotoxicity. The no-observed-adverse-effect level was 0.5 mg/kg body weight in mice and rats and 0.75 mg/kg body weight in hamsters. Endrin did not induce reproductive effects in rats over three generations when given at a dose of 2 mg/kg of diet (about 0.1 mg/kg body weight).

A number of the metabolites of endrin have similar or higher acute toxicities than the parent compound. The transformation product, delta-ketoendrin, is less toxic than endrin, but 12-ketoendrin is considered to be the most toxic metabolite of endrin in mammals, with an oral LD_{50} in rats of 0.8–1.1 mg/kg body weight.

1.1.5   Effects on human beings

Several episodes of fatal and non-fatal accidental and suicidal poisoning have occurred. Cases of acute non-fatal intoxication due to accidental over-exposure were observed in workers in an endrin manufacturing plant. The oral dose that causes death has been estimated to be approximately 10 mg/kg body weight; the single oral dose that causes convulsions was estimated to be 0.25–1.0 mg/kg body weight.

The primary site of action of endrin is the central nervous system. Exposure of humans to a toxic dose may lead within a few hours to such signs and symptoms of intoxication as excitability and convulsions, and death may follow within 2–12 h after exposure if appropriate treatment is not administered immediately. Recovery from non-fatal poisoning is rapid and complete.

Endrin does not accumulate in the human body to any significant degree. No long-term adverse effects were reported in 232 occupationally exposed workers (length of exposure, 4–27 years) under medical supervision (observation time, 4–29 years). The only effect observed was indirect evidence of a reversible stimulation of drug metabolizing enzymes.

Endrin was detected in virtually none of a large number of samples of adipose tissue, blood, and breast milk analysed in many countries. The Task Group attributed the absence of endrin in human samples to the low exposure of the general population to this pesticide and to its rapid metabolism.

Endrin was detected in blood (at up to 450 µg/litre) and in adipose tissue (at 89.5 mg/kg) in cases of fatal accidental poisoning. No endrin was found in workers under normal circumstances. The threshold level of endrin in blood, below which no sign or symptom of intoxication occurs, has been estimated to be 50–100 µg/litre. The half-life of endrin in blood may be in the order of 24 h.

Summary and evaluation; conclusions; recommendations

1.2 Conclusions

Endrin is an insecticide with high acute toxicity. It may cause severe poisoning in cases of over-exposure caused by careless handling during its manufacture and use or by consumption of contaminated food. The general public is exposed to endrin mainly as its residues in food; however, the reported intake of endrin is generally far below the acceptable daily intake established by FAO/WHO. Such exposures should not constitute a health hazard to the general population. When good work practices, hygiene measures, and safety precautions are enforced, endrin is unlikely to present a hazard to exposed workers.

It is clear that uncontrolled discharges of endrin during its manufacture, formulation, and use can result in acute environmental problems associated with its high toxicity. The effects on wildlife of its agricultural use are less clear, although fish and fish-eating birds are at risk from surface run-off. Declines in the populations of some avian species have been associated with the presence of high levels of residues of various organochlorines in the tissues of adults and in eggs. Endrin has been measured in some of these species; however, it is very difficult to separate the effects of the different organochlorines present.

1.3 Recommendations

1. Endrin should not be used unless it is indispensable and only when no less toxic alternative is available.

2. For the health and welfare of workers and the general population, the handling and application of endrin should be entrusted only to competently supervised, well-trained operators who will follow adequate safety measures and apply endrin according to good agricultural practices.

3. The manufacture, formulation, agricultural use, and disposal of endrin should be managed carefully to minimize contamination of the environment, particularly surface water.

4. People exposed regularly to endrin should undergo periodic health evaluations.

5. Epidemiological studies of exposed worker populations should be continued.

6. In countries where endrin is still used, food should be monitored for endrin residues.

7. If the use of endrin continues, more information should be obtained on the presence, ultimate fate, and toxicity of 12-ketoendrin and delta-ketoendrin.

2. IDENTITY, PHYSICAL AND CHEMICAL PROPERTIES, ANALYTICAL METHODS

2.1 Identity

CAS chemical name: (1aα,2β,2aβ,3α,6α,6aβ,7β,7aα)-3,4,5,6,9.9-hexachloro 1a,2,2a,3, 6, 6a,7,7a-octahydro-2,7:3,6-dimethanonaphth[2,3-b]oxirene (9CI-CAS)

Former CAS chemical name: 1,2,3,4,10,10-hexachloro-6,7-epoxy-1,4,4a,5,6,7,8,8a-octahydro-1,4-*endo,endo*-5,8-dimethanonaphthalene

IUPAC chemical name: 1R,4S,4aS,5S,6S,7R,8R,8aR)-1,2,3,4,10,10-hexachloro-1,4,4a,5,6,7,8,8a-octahydro-6,7-epoxy-1,4:5,8- dimethanonaphthalene

Chemical structure:

Endrin is the *endo,endo* stereoisomer of dieldrin
Empirical formula: $C_{12}H_8Cl_6O$
Relative molecular mass: 380.93
Common name: Endrin
CAS registry number: 72-20-8
RTECS registry number: I01575000
Synonyms: Endrex, Experimental Insecticide 269, Hexadrin, Nendrin, NCI-COO157, ENT17251, OMS 197, and Mendrin
Trade name: Endrin

Purity: Not less than 92%. Impurities include dieldrin (0.42%), aldrin (0.03%), isodrin (0.73%), endrin half-cage ketone (1.57%), endrin aldehyde (0.05%), and heptachloronorbornene (0.09%) (Donoso et al., 1979).

2.2 Physical and chemical properties

Table 1. Physical and chemical properties of endrin

Physical state	Crystalline solid
Colour	White to light-tan
Odour	Mild chemical
Melting-point	226–230 °C (decomposes at above 245 °C)
Flash-point	None (dry powder is non-flammable, but commercial solutions contain inflammable liquids with flash-points as low as 27 °C)
Explosion limits	Non-explosive
Specific gravity (density)	1.64 g/ml at 20 °C
Vapour pressure	2.7×10^{-7} mmHg at 25 °C (36 µPa at 25 °C)
Solubility in water	Practically insoluble (0.23 mg/litre at 25 °C)
Solubility in organic solvents	Sparingly soluble in alcohol and petroleum hydrocarbons; moderately soluble in aliphatic hydrocarbons; and quite soluble in solvents such as acetone, benzene, carbon tetrachloride, and xylene
Log P octanol/water partition coefficient	5.34

Stability: Technical-grade endrin is stable in storage at ambient temperatures. Endrin is stable in formulations with basic reagents, alkaline oxidizing agents, emulsifiers,

Identity, physical and chemical properties, analytical methods

wetting agents, and solvents. It isomerizes under the influence of ultraviolet light. It reacts with concentrated mineral acids, acid catalysts, acid oxidizing agents and active metals. When mixed with certain catalytically active carriers, endrin tends to decompose; however, most active dust carriers can be deactivated by the addition of hexamethylenetetramine and form stable mixtures with endrin. When heated to above 200 °C, endrin undergoes molecular rearrangements to form delta-ketoendrin, a compound that is less active as an insecticide (IARC, 1974; Donoso et al., 1979).

2.3 Conversion factors

1 ppm = 16 mg/m^3 at 20 °C
1 mg/m^3 = 0.063 ppm at 20 °C

2.4 Analytical methods

Most of the analytical procedures used since the early 1960s have been based on the following steps:
  (i)   extraction using a suitable solvent;
  (ii) clean-up by liquid/liquid partition followed by column chromatography;
  (iii) further separation from co-extractives by gas chromatography (GC); and
  (iv) quantification using an electron-capture, coulometric, or Hall electrolytic detector

General procedures based on these steps are not specific for endrin; therefore, its identity must be confirmed in environmental samples. This can be achieved by chemical derivatization and mass spectrometry (Chau & Cochrane, 1969, 1971; Belisle et al., 1972; Chau, 1974; Safe & Hutzinger, 1979).

Roos et al. (1987) used size exclusion chromatography to clean-up pesticides after extraction with ethyl acetate from fish oils, animal fat, cereals, vegetables, fruit, and liver. The recoveries of endrin were 90–95%, at a limit of detection of 0.02 mg/kg. This method was found to be adequate for screening and requires only 15% of the amount of solvents normally used.

Gübeli & Clerc (1988) described a relatively simple gas–liquid chromatography method for the detection and approximate quantification of chlorinated pesticides in ethanolic extracts of medicinal plants (tinctures). The method was based on extraction with hexane and capillary GC/^{63}Ni-electron-capture detection. The limit of detection for endrin was 0.005 mg/kg with a recovery of 77.5%.

Suzuki et al. (1974) separated many pesticides from extracts of crops and soil into different groups by column chromatography prior to thin-layer chromatography to obtain systematic identification and determination. Silica gel was used for the column chromatography and for the thin-layer plates; glass columns packed with different absorbents were used for GC separation. Determination was done using electron-capture detection with a ^{63}Ni source.

To improve the separation by heat of 28 organochlorine insecticides, including endrin, using gas–liquid chromatography with electron capture detection, Suzuki & Morimoto (1986) tested three chemically bonded, fused silica capillary columns. The column prepared with OV-17 performed best. The method was used with minimal clean-up and gave good results in the analysis of extracts of several soil samples, avoiding the disadvantages of low resolution of peaks in packed columns, handling of glass capillary columns and the high cost of GC–mass spectrometry systems.

Kiang & Grob (1986) developed a screening procedure for the determination of 49 pollutants of high priority, including endrin, in soil or sludge. Methylene chloride at two pH values was used in the extraction procedure, which was followed by capillary GC. No clean-up procedure was carried out. Separation and identification were performed with a GC–mass spectrometry system involving a 30-m fused silica column; a 60-m column was used for quantification. Recovery of endrin from soil in the base–neutral extract was $92 \pm 14\%$ from 2.04 mg/kg but only $70 \pm 8\%$ from 20.4 mg/kg.

Japenga et al. (1987) described a rapid clean-up procedure for the simultaneous determination of groups of micropollutants in sediment. The samples were pretreated with acid, mixed with silica, and extracted on a Soxhlet column with a mixture of benzene and hexane. Humic substances and elemental sulfur were removed by passing the extract through a chromatographic column containing basic alumina on which sodium sulfite and sodium hydroxide were absorbed. After silica fractionation, the concentrations of polycyclic aromatic hydrocarbons, polychlorinated biphenyls, and chlorinated pesticides were determined by GC. The recovery of endrin was reported to fluctuate between 93 and 103%.

The efficiency of clean-up with sulfuric acid and confirmation with potassium hydroxide–ethanol hydrolysis was studied for 22 organochlorine pesticides and polychlorinated biphenyls in water samples (Hernandez et al., 1987); analysis was by GC/electron-capture detection, and the pesticides were extracted by partition with 15% diethyl ether in hexane. After clean-up with sulfuric acid, only 4.9% of the endrin was recovered; however, with the potassium hydroxide–ethanol treatment, 97–100% was recovered, depending on the endrin concentration and the length of treatment.

Method 8080 of the US Environmental Protection Agency (EPA) (Manual, SW-846) was evaluated in a single laboratory study by Lopez-Avila et al. (1988). Since the Florisil clean-up procedure recommended does not separate organochlorine pesticides from polychlorinated biphenyls, GC analysis on a packed column may result in false identifications; therefore, silica gel was substituted for Florisil, a capillary glass column was used instead of the packed column, and a procedure to remove elemental sulfur incorporated. Detection limits for liquid matrices ranged from 0.02 to 0.09 µg/litre for organochlorine pesticides; for solid matrices, a range of 1–6 µg/kg was found. The recovery of endrin in liquid waste was up to 102% at a spiked concentration of 1.0 µg, but for a sandy loam soil it varied from 47 to 74%.

Donahue et al. (1988) compared two techniques for quantifying environmental contaminants in human serum: peak area matching and linear regression. No statistically significant difference was seen in the results obtained by these two methods when the concentration of chlorinated pesticides was > 0.5 µg/litre.

The sampling and determination of endrin in air were described in detail by NIOSH (1989).

A method for determining residues of the metabolite *anti*-12-hydroxy-endrin, present as the ß-glucuronide, in urine was described by Baldwin & Hutson (1980). Following oxidation with sodium metaperiodate and hydrolysis with a mild base, the metabolite is determined by gas–liquid chromatography with electron-capture detection.

Polychlorinated biphenyls and 21 chlorinated pesticides, including endrin, were analysed in samples of water, soil, and sediment in six laboratories using uniform calibration solutions, analytical methods, and special software operating on minicomputers to control the operation of the mass spectrometer. The results obtained for solid samples with four combinations of methods for extraction and clean-up were compared; although no combination was optimal for all samples, shaker and sonicator extraction, both with Florisil clean-up, gave the best results. Several factors that affected the quality of the results were identified, including errors in computation and transcription and inadequate review of data (Alford-Stevens et al., 1988).

Seventeen laboratories participated in an international comparison of analyses for organochlorine compounds (Holden, 1970). The results for endrin, summarized in Table 2, were more variable than those for other insecticides. In an inter-laboratory collaborative study reported by a Committee of the Ministry of Agriculture, Fisheries, and Food of the United Kingdom (Anon., 1979) for the determination of endrin in pork fat (fortified to 0.019 mg/kg), the mean recovery in 11 laboratories was 84%, but the range was 5–131%.

Table 2. Results for endrin of an inter-laboratory study of the analysis of organochlorine compounds (Holden, 1970)

Type of sample	No. of laboratories with results for endrin	Mean concentration (mg/litre or mg/kg)	Standard deviation	Coefficient of variation (%)	Range
Solution in hexane[a]	17	5.929[b]	1.01	17.1	4.9–8.2
Cod liver oil	14	0.02	–	–	ND[c]–0.20[d]
Chicken egg	16	0.136	0.073	54	0.07–0.3[e]
Sprat	14	0.132	0.039	29	0.09[f]–0.21

[a] Containing endrin and five other organochlorine insecticides
[b] True (nominal, fortified) value, 7.05 mg/litre
[c] Twelve laboratories reported no detectable residue
[d] Value reported to be suspect
[e] Excluding one laboratory that reported suspected presence of endrin
[f] Excluding one laboratory that reported a 'trace' of endrin

Table 3. Methods for the analysis of endrin

Sample type	Extraction	Clean-up	Detection and quantification[a]	Recovery (%)	Limit of detection	Reference
Adipose tissue	Acetone:hexane (15:85 v/v)	Fractionation by gel permeation chromatography with methylene chloride–cyclohexane Florisil column	Capillary column gas chromatography columns of different polarity, GC–MS	> 100		Lebel & Williams (1986)
Air	Hexylene glycol/Greenburg Smith impinger; alumina column	Florisil column	GLC/ECD	77	0.1 ng/m^3	Stanley et al. (1971)
Air	Toluene	–	GLC/ECD (^{63}Ni)	–	0.02 µg/sample	NIOSH (1989)
Water	Hexane:ethyl ether	–	GLC/ECD	65–97	0.002 µg/litre	Lichtenberg et al. (1970)
Soil/sediment	Acetone:hexane	Alumina column	GLC/ECD	83	0.1 µg/kg	Goerlitz & Law (1974)
Soil/sediment	Acetone:petroleum ether	Alumina column	GLC/ECD	90	0.01 mg/kg	Wegman & Hofstee (1982)

Table 3 (contd)

Sample type	Extraction	Clean-up	Detection and quantification [a]	Recovery	Limit of detection	Reference
Soil/sediment	Hexane	Alumina/silver nitrate + silica gel column	GLC/ECD	–	0.01 mg/kg	McIntyre & Lester (1984)
Crops	Hexane:isopropanol; or acetonitrile	Carbon absorption (Nuchar C-190N)	GLC/ECD	93–107	–	Kathpal & Dewan (1975)
Fatty foods, vegetable oils, fish oils	Hexane:acetone	Alumina column	GLC/ECD	68–100	5-10 µg/kg	Telling et al. (1977)
Viscera	Diethyl ether	Celite column	GLC/ECD	72–92	–	Kurhekar et al. (1975)
Birds' brain samples	Petroleum ether: ethyl ether	Florisil column	GLC/ECD	70	0.05 mg/kg	Ludke (1976)
Cows' milk	Diethyl ether: hexane + ether	Silica gel	GLC/ECD	90	0.0001 mg/kg	Baldwin et al. (1976)
Hens' eggs (yolks)	Hexane:acetone	Silica gel	GLC/ECD	76	0.05 mg/kg	Baldwin et al. (1976)

Table 3 (contd)

Sample type	Extraction	Clean-up	Detection and quantification[a]	Recovery	Limit of detection	Reference
Crops, soil, milk, animal tissues	Hydrocarbon solvent (Skellysolve B) + isopropanol	Florisil:Celite + magnesia column, after alkaline hydrolysis, if appropriate	Reduction with metallic sodium; phenyl azide colorimetry	75–100	1 mg/kg	Terriere (1964)

[a] GC–MS, gas chromatography–mass spectometry; GLC–ECD, gas-liquid chromatography–electron capture detection

Thier & Stijve (1986) reported a comparative study among 53 laboratories in Switzerland on the analysis of a vegetable fat spiked with 13 organochlorine and five organophosphorus compounds. Endrin was present at a concentration of 0.08 mg/kg and was identified by 77% of the laboratories.

Some of the methods that are used for the analysis of endrin are summarized in Table 3; the estimates given of the accuracy of the procedures and the limits of detection refer to the specific investigations and are not absolute values. The percentage recoveries are an indication of the accuracy of the methods; the precision of individual method is of interest particularly in regard to inter-laboratory comparisons.

The many publications on specific procedures are reviewed in the Codex Alimentarius Commission publication *Recommendations for Methods of Analysis of Pesticide Residues*, CAC/PR8-1986 (FAO/WHO, 1986a). That review lists 14 individual publications; it also lists the following compendia of methods, which may be consulted.

— *Official Methods of Analysis of the Association of Official Analytical Chemists*, 14th Edition, 1984
— *Pesticide Analytical Manual*, Washington DC, Food and Drug Administration
— *Manual on Analytical Methods for Pesticide Residues in Foods*, Ottawa, Health Protection Branch, Health and Welfare Canada, 1985
— *Methodensammlung zur Rückstandsanalytik von Pflanzenschutzmitteln* (Methods for Analysing Residues of Plant Protection Agents), Weinheim, Verlag Chemie GmbH, 1984
— *Chemistry Laboratory Guidebook*, Washington DC, US Department of Agriculture

Whatever procedure is adopted should be carried out following the requirements of the Codex Alimentarius Commission publication *Codex Guidelines on Good Laboratory Practice in Pesticide Residue Analysis*, CAC/PR7-1984 (FAO/WHO, 1984).

3. SOURCES OF HUMAN AND ENVIRONMENTAL EXPOSURE

3.1 Natural occurrence

Endrin does not occur naturally.

3.2 Man-made sources

3.2.1 Production levels and processes, uses

Endrin is a foliar insecticide which acts against a wide range of agricultural pests at doses of the active material of 0.2–0.5 kg/ha. It has a broad spectrum of control and is particularly effective against Lepidoptera. It is used mainly on cotton but also against pests of rice, sugar cane, maize, and other crops. It is also used as a rodenticide (IARC, 1974). An endrin emulsion of 2% killed 40% of *Achatina fulica* snails, an agricultural pest, in India (Singh, 1988).

A general indication of the possible uses of endrin can be derived from the maximal residue limits recommended by FAO/WHO (1986b; see section 10).

3.2.1.1 World production figures

Endrin was developed by J. Hyman & Co. and licensed to be manufactured by Shell International Chemical Co. and Velsicol Chemical Co. in 1950 (Thompson, 1976). It was made in the USA by Shell and Velsicol and in the Netherlands by Shell. Its use has been banned in many countries and severely restricted in others (Donoso et al., 1979; Gips, 1987; Pearce, 1987). Shell discontinued manufacture of endrin in 1982; it is still manufactured in Mexico.

Whetstone (1964) estimated that 2.3–4.5 million kg of endrin were sold in the USA in 1962. Imports of endrin into Japan in 1970 were 72 000 kg. The annual quantities of endrin that were used in paddy rice production in Bali over the period 1963–72 varied from 171 to 10 700 kg (Machbub et al., 1988). After 1972, endrin was no longer used.

3.2.1.2 Manufacturing process

Endrin is produced by condensing vinyl chloride with hexachlorocyclopentadiene, dehydrochlorinating the adduct, and subsequent reaction with cyclopentadiene to form isodrin, which is epoxidized by peracetic or perbenzoic acid (Whetstone, 1964). The intermediate isodrin can be manufactured via 1,2,3,4,7,7-hexachloronorbornadiene (US EPA, 1985).

4. ENVIRONMENTAL TRANSPORT, DISTRIBUTION, AND TRANSFORMATION

4.1 Transport and distribution between media

4.1.1 *Air*

Endrin can enter the air by volatilization, evaporation, and aerial drift during application, and as a vapour from manufacturing and formulating plants. Most studies showed rapid volatilization following application to soils and crops, the extent of vaporization depending upon a large number of factors, including soil organic matter, moisture content, air humidity, air flow, and surface area of plants (Donoso et al., 1979).

4.1.2 *Water*

Endrin can reach surface water by several routes, including effluents and waste disposal from endrin manufacturing and formulating plants and careless aerial application, but by far the most important route of contamination is surface run-off from soil and crops. Run-off is affected by numerous, complex factors, such as intensity of precipitation, irrigation practices, soil permeability, topographic relief, organic content of the soil, and the degree of vegetative cover. Soils of low permeability and low organic content allow copious run-off after heavy precipitation (Donoso et al., 1979). Contamination of surface water by industrial effluents and careless practices and disposal (such as washing of drums and spray equipment in streams) results in regional effects.

In 1961, studies were conducted in the Bayou Yokely basin in Louisiana, USA, where 3300 acres (1335 ha) of sugar-cane were treated with nearly 2000 lb (907 kg) of endrin between June and August. Of 18 water samples taken between April and November, six contained endrin at levels of 0.001–0.36 µg/litre, with an average of 0.1 µg/litre. In 1964, the area was treated with 1200 lb (544 kg) of endrin, and the pattern of residues was the same. The mean residue levels in samples taken in September were 0.44 µg/litre in grab samples and 0.53 µg/litre in carbon adsorption samples; after three months, the average levels were 0.03 and 0.04 µg/litre, respectively. Sediment samples contained 165 µg/kg; after three months, this level had decreased to 70 µg/kg (Lauer et al., 1966).

Another, less important source of water contamination is run-off from endrin-coated seeds. Marston et al. (1969) found that although approximately 11% of the initial amount was washed off by water under laboratory conditions, in field conditions the loss was smaller. The total amount detected in the watershed 6 days after aerial application of endrin-coated seed was 0.12% of the applied dose. The highest concentration found in the water was 0.07 µg/litre.

A third possible source of contamination is fall-out by precipitation in the form of rain and snow, but the measured levels are negligible (see section 5.1.3.2).

4.1.3 Soil

The major source of endrin in soil is from direct application to soil and crops. The amount of endrin that reaches the soil depends on the type of crop and the method of application. The fate of endrin in soil determines the degree to which the rest of the environment (water and atmosphere) is contaminated. In soil, endrin can be retained, transported, or degraded, depending on a large number of interrelated factors (Donoso et al., 1979). When endrin was applied to tall, dense crops such as tobacco, no residue appeared in the soil; when it was applied to soil, the amount that remained depended on the retentive ability of the soil. Although endrin has strong absorptive properties in soils such as clay and sandy loam, limited residues were found. Far greater retention was found in soils with a high organic content, in which it was adsorbed quickly and was difficult to remove. The degree to which endrin was retained in the soil depended not only on the soil type but on numerous other factors such as volatilization, leaching, wind erosion, surface run-off, and crop uptake (Harris et al., 1966). In general, the persistence of endrin is highly dependent upon local conditions, and residue levels can range from traces to milligrams per kilogram. Its half-life in soil can be as long as 12 years (Donoso et al., 1979).

The factors that affect the degree to which endrin is retained in soil (Donoso et al., 1979) can be generalized as follows:

(a) Endrin appears to be less persistent if it is applied to the soil surface or to crops rather than being mixed into the soil.
(b) Volatilization and photodecomposition are the primary routes for the disappearance of endrin from soil surfaces.
(c) Microbial degradation of endrin occurs anaerobically and is accelerated by conditions such as flooding and soil depth.

(d) Soil cultivation and crop rotation accelerate the dissipation of endrin.

(e) When the percentage of organic matter is high, as in muck-soils, the persistence of eldrin is greater. In sandy soils, volatilization is high and persistence is low.

4.1.4 Soil–plants

River and basin sediment was brought on land near Rotterdam, the Netherlands, after dredging. Once the sediment had settled for several years, the land was used for agriculture. Some of the sediment came from a basin near a pesticide manufacturing plant and was contaminated with many organochlorine hydrocarbons, including the pesticides hexachlorobenzene, aldrin, dieldrin, and endrin. The mean concentration of endrin in the sediment of the basin near the plant (expressed in mg/kg on a dry weight basis) was 0.48 (range, 0.01-2.6) in 1976 and 0.59 (< 0.01-3.6) in 1977. In crops, the concentration of endrin ranged from none detected to 0.06 mg/kg of product; in carrots, however, levels up to 0.73 mg/kg were found (Wegman et al., 1981).

4.2 Abiotic degradation

When endrin was heated to above 200 °C, as can occur during gas–liquid chromatography at 230 °C, the molecule was isomerized to a ketone, delta-ketoendrin (*1*, Fig. 1) and an aldehyde (*3*). A minor product of the thermal rearrangement was an isomeric alcohol (*4*). Endrin is also transformed to delta-ketoendrin (*1*) under acid-catalysed conditions (Phillips et al., 1962).

Irradiation with ultraviolet light for 48 h also results in rearrangement to this ketone (37%) and, to a much lesser extent, to the aldehyde (9%) (Rosen et al., 1966; Plimmer, 1972; Mukerjee, 1985). Endrin underwent a photolytic reaction in hexane and in cyclohexane after irradiation at 253.7 and 300 nm, resulting in a half-cage ketone, pentachloro photoproduct (*2*), in 80% yield. This photolytic product has also been identified in the field and was found to be highly resistant to oxidation and reduction (Plimmer, 1972; Zabik et al., 1971; Mukerjee, 1985). When an acetone solution of endrin was irradiated with light from a mercury lamp in a quartz cell for 24 h, three metabolites were formed by the loss of one chlorine atom from the initially produced delta-ketoendrin; one of these was compound 2 (Dureja et al., 1987).

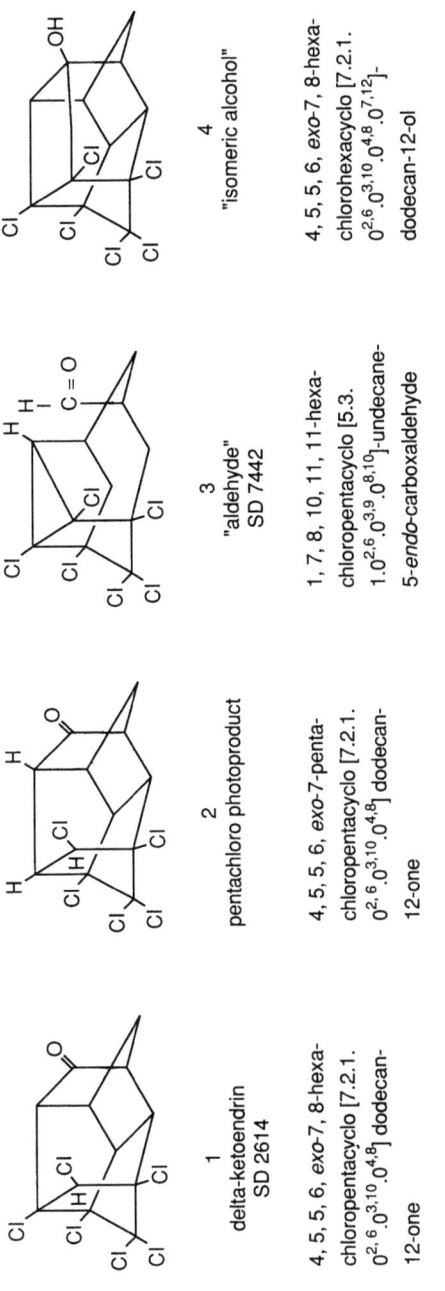

Fig. 1. Structural formulae and chemical names of thermal and photolytic conversion products of endrin

Environmental transport, distribution, and transformation

Endrin has been reported to isomerize to delta-ketoendrin during 5 years' storage in the dark at room temperature (Plimmer, 1972).

In sunlight, mainly the ketone is formed (Soto & Deichmann, 1967; Rosen, 1972); approximately 50% isomerization to the ketone took place within 7 ± 2 days with exposure to intense summer sun (Burton & Pollard, 1974).

The photochemical products are important as terminal residues: delta-ketoendrin was found on cotton plants and on cabbage and apple leaves after application of endrin (Plimmer, 1971; Mukerjee, 1985).

4.3 Biotransformation

The mechanisms by which endrin is removed from the environment include photodecomposition and bacterial degradation. These factors and their effects on the persistence of endrin have been reviewed by the US Environmental Protection Agency (Donoso et al., 1979).

4.3.1 Biodegradation

Microbial degradation of endrin depends on the presence of an appropriate microbial species and suitable soil conditions; it occurs under anaerobic conditions (Donoso et al., 1979). Biodegradation is aided by fungi and bacteria such as *Trichoderma*, *Pseudomonas*, and *Bacillus*. The major transformation product is delta-ketoendrin (Patil et al., 1970).

About 150 isolates from various soil samples were screened to investigate the role of these microorganisms in degrading endrin; 25 of the 150 isolates were active. At least seven metabolites were found, but conversion of endrin into the ketoendrin was common throughout (Matsumura et al., 1971).

4.3.2 Bioaccumulation and biomagnification

The bioconcentration factors cited below are simple ratios of the exposure concentration and the concentration in organic tissues. They should be used with caution as indicators of bioaccumulation potential: a high bioconcentration factor can represent little uptake of a low concentration, and a low bioconcentration factor can be found with considerable uptake of a high concentration. The bioconcentration factor should therefore always be cited with the pertinent exposure concentration of endrin.

Soil invertebrates such as slugs and earthworms had bioconcentration factors of 14 to 103. Bioconcentration factors in a number of aquatic organisms are given in Table 4. These ratios differ extensively between different types of aquatic organisms. Bioconcentration factors of 140 to 222 were found for four blue-green algae (*Microcystis aeruginosa, Anabaena cylindrica, Scenedesmus quadricauda,* and an *Oedogonium* species) after 7 days' exposure to endrin at a concentration of 1 mg/litre of water(Vance & Drummond, 1969). In a study of the accumulation of endrin in stoneflies (*Pteronarcys dorsata*) exposed to 0.03, 0.07, and 0.15 µg/litre of water, the bioconcentration factor ranged from 1130 to 348, decreasing with increasing water concentrations over the 28-day exposure period (Anderson & DeFoe, 1980). In bullheads (*Ictalurus melas*), the bioconcentration factor was 3700 after exposure for 4 days to 0.60 µg/litre and 6200 after exposure for 7 days to 0.26 µg/litre (Anderson & DeFoe, 1980). The bioconcentration factors for endrin in sub-adults of leopard frogs (*Rana sphenocephala*) exposed to 0.01, 0.012, 0.016, 0.022, and 0.030 mg/litre were 71.4, 34.4, 51.8, 59.4, and 94.3, respectively. Sub-adults exposed to 0.01, 0.012, and 0.016 mg/litre for 96 h and sacrificed 60 h later had bioconcentration factors of 6.1, 4.8, and 1.2, respectively (Hall & Swineford, 1980), indicating a relatively rapid elimination of residues.

In daphnids and molluscs, a direct linear relationship was found between the logarithm of the equilibrium bioconcentration factor (and the reciprocal clearance rate constant) and the log P octanol/water partition coefficient for non-degradable, lipophilic compounds with partition coefficients ranging from 2 to 6. This relationship permits calculation of the times required for equilibrium and for significant bioconcentration of lipophilic chemicals, which were found to be shorter for molluscs than for daphnids. The equilibrium biotic concentration for both molluscs and daphnids decreased with increasing chemical hydrophobicity. The relationship between the bioconcentration factor and log P octanol/water partition coefficient was linear for compounds that did not attain equilibrium within a finite exposure time (Hawker & Connell, 1986).

In a study of the bioaccumulation of endrin from food by lobsters (*Homarus americanus*), endrin dissolved in methanol was added to sea water, and mussel tissue was soaked in the solution for 2 h to provide

Table 4. Bioconcentration factors for endrin in aquatic species

Species	Concentration of endrin in water (µg/litre)	Length of exposure	Bioconcentration factor	Reference
Clam (*Mercenaria mercenaria*)	1	5 days	480	Duke & Dumas (1974)
Mussel (*Hyridella australis*)	10	24 days	38	Ryan et al. (1972)
Eastern oyster (*Crassostrea virginica*)	0.05	7 day	2780	Mason & Rowe (1976)
Water flea (*Daphnia magna*)	1.0	1 day	2600	Metcalf et al. (1973)
Fathead minnow (*Pimephales promelas*)	0.015	–	10 000	Mount & Putnicki (1966)
Spot (*Leiostomus xanthurus*)	0.05	8 months	1340	Lowe (1966)
Flag fish (*Jordanella floridae*)	0.3 0.21 0.29 0.39	– 15 days	10 000 7 900 18 400 7 100	Hermanutz (1974) Hermanutz et al. (1985)
Mosquito larvae (*Culex ipiensquinque fasciatus*)	1.0	1 day	2 100	Metcalf et al. (1973)
Mosquito fish (*Gambusia affinis*)	1.0	1 day	800	Metcalf et al. (1973)
Channel catfish (*Ictalurus punctatus*)	0.5	5–19	400–760	Argyle et al. (1973)

a concentration of endrin of 4.7 mg/kg wet weight. Lobsters were fed the prepared food every other day for 2 weeks, and excretion was followed for an additional 4 weeks during which time the lobsters were fed uncontaminated tissue. Liver and muscle were analysed from two or three lobsters sampled after feedings 1, 2, 3, 5, and 7, and from one or two lobsters sampled during the excretion phase at 1, 2, and 4 weeks. The concentration of endrin reached a maximum of 1.95 mg/kg wet weight in the liver after 2 weeks of feeding; this level declined by about 65% after 4 weeks of excretion. The time to 90% equilibrium (uptake) was 15 weeks, and the time to 50% clearance (excretion) was 4 weeks (McLeese et al., 1980).

Bluegill sunfish (*Lepomis macrochirus*) exposed to water containing ^{14}C-labelled endrin at 1 µg/litre at temperatures of 20–22 °C rapidly absorbed the radioactivity, and, within 48 h, 91% of the radioactive endrin had been taken up (6% was lost by volatilization from a control tank without fish). Within 8 days after the fish had been replaced in clean water, less than 15% of the absorbed label had been eliminated; for three fish left for a longer period, the half-life of loss was about 4 weeks, the loss curve being linear (Sundershan & Khan, 1980). Endrin accumulated rapidly in the tissues of channel catfish (*Ictalurus punctatus*) exposed to nominal concentrations of 0.04, 0.4, or 4.0 mg/kg of diet for 198 days. After that time, all groups were fed an endrin-free diet. Endrin was not detected 28 days later in fish that had received 0.04 or 0.4 mg/kg, and the level in the group that had received 4.0 mg/kg decreased to 0.011 mg/kg of tissue in 28 days and was below the limit of detection within 41 days (Argyle et al., 1973). Similar results were obtained for *Leiostomus xantharus* exposed to 0.05 µg/litre of water: at the end of the study at 5 months, a residue level of 78 µg/kg tissue was found, and no endrin was detected in fish after 18 days in uncontaminated water (Lowe, 1966). Endrin thus seems to disappear rapidly from tissues. In 20 *Tilapia zilli* (Alexandria strain) fry (3.36 cm, 825 mg) exposed to 0.025 µg/litre (one-tenth of the 96-h LC_{50}) for 28 days, the total content of endrin was 327.4, 167.4, 297.6, 446.5, and 595.4 µg/kg after 4, 7, 14, 21, and 28 days, respectively (El-Sebae, 1987).

Sheepshead minnow (*Cyprinodon variegatus*) were exposed for 23 weeks to endrin at levels of 0.027–0.72 µg/litre of water, from the embryonic stage through hatching until adulthood and spawning (see section 7.2.2.2). Four-week-old juvenile fish accumulated 2500 times the concentration in the water, adults, 6400 times, and their eggs, 5700 times (Hansen et al., 1977).

Environmental transport, distribution, and transformation

The transfer of endrin through the food chain lichen–reindeer–humans was studied in the northern part of Sweden by analysing lichen (*Cladonia alpestris*), a major food source for reindeer during the winter, together with samples of tissues from reindeer, which are eaten in considerable quantities by Lapps. One 4-year-old reindeer was slaughtered in 1979 and a 3-year-old in 1981, and muscle and liver were taken for analysis. The annual uptake by reindeer was 2.0 mg. The average level of endrin in lichen was 1.91 (range, 1.27–2.78) µg/kg; 1.45 and 2.4 µg/kg were found in the muscle samples from the two reindeer and 0.55 and 0.72 µg/kg in liver. The calculated transfer of endrin from lichen to reindeer was 0.7%. The estimated annual consumption of reindeer muscle by Lapps was 70 kg for males and 32 kg for women; consumption of liver was 3 and 1.1 kg, respectively. The annual intake of endrin was thus 30.3 µg for males and 13.8 µg for females (Villeneuve et al., 1985).

5. ENVIRONMENTAL LEVELS AND HUMAN EXPOSURE

Many of the data reported in this chapter are measurements taken at a time when endrin was used much more widely than at present or with little control or restriction. They are therefore a reflection of a historical situation in many countries. These data are included in the document as an indication of the result of indiscriminate use and disposal of endrin. Data from countries where endrin may still be used are scarce or unavailable.

5.1 Environmental levels

The levels of residues associated with the use of endrin in agriculture or with the discharge of industrial effluents containing endrin are summarized in Tables 5–9; the levels of residues less easily associated with specific uses or discharges are given in Table 10.

5.1.1 Air

A critical summary of studies on the atmospheric levels of pesticides in the USA, e.g., in community air, was made by Donoso et al. (1979). Some of their conclusions are worth repeating: "Endrin concentrations are highest in the atmosphere over agricultural areas and probably reach their peak levels during the pesticide use season. Of all urban communities those surrounded by farmlands run the highest chance of atmospheric contamination. Urban communities far removed from agricultural areas are unlikely to experience significant contamination." The maximum level of endrin in air, 58.5 ng/m^3, was found in a rural town in an agricultural area in the south of the USA, but the normal weekly variation was between 0.8 and 6.5 ng/m^3 (Stanley et al., 1971). In a later study of the same town, the average annual atmospheric levels were 3.2 ng/m^3 in 1972, 2.3 ng/m^3 in 1973, and 5.3 ng/m^3 in 1974, with the highest levels in August; in 1974, this was 27.2 ng/m^3 (Arthur et al., 1976). The results of a national monitoring programme for pesticides in the air of various states of the USA showed the occasional presence of endrin over agricultural areas at levels of the same order of magnitude: mean of positive samples (8%), 2.6 ng/m^3, with a maximum value of 19.2 ng/m^3 (Kutz et al., 1976).

Endrin was not found in rain-water collected at different location in the United Kingdom, using a method with a detection level of 1 ng/litre of

Table 5. Concentrations of endrin in organisms collected in the Netherlands, 1965–71

Place and period	Type of sample	No. of samples[a]	Concentration (mg/kg) Mean	Concentration (mg/kg) Range[b]	Comments	Reference
Coast 1965	Mussel (*Mystilus edulis*); composites of flesh	22	0.029	0.009–0.056	Composites of 25 mussels from 22 sampling stations	Koeman (1971)
Netherlands 1965	Fish, 3 species; whole body	103	0.13	0.07–0.45		Koeman et al. (1967)
1966	Fish, 3 species; whole body Sandwich tern (*Sterna sandvincensis*)	37	0.10	0.07–0.29	Food of the sandwich tern	
1965	Liver	8	0.23	0.07–0.80	Shot or killed	
1965–66	Liver	25	0.49	0.10–1.3	Found dead	
1965–66	Egg	33	0.19	0.08–0.36		
Wadden Sea 1969	Mussel (2 species); composites of flesh	20/4	LD	LD	Limit of detection, 0.005 mg/kg	Koeman (1971)

Table 5. (contd)

Place and period	Type of sample	No. of samples[a]	Concentration (mg/kg) Mean	Concentration (mg/kg) Range[b]	Comments	Reference
Coast 1970	Mussel (*Mytilus edulis*); composites of flesh	199/8	< 0.016	LD–0.024		Koeman (1971)
Wadden Sea 1969–70	Zooplankton (marine)	1	LD	LD		Koeman (1971)
	Shrimp (*Crangon vulgaris*)	50/1	LD	LD		
	Marine fish (4 species); composites of whole body	37/5	0.014	0.008–0.034		
1967	Freshwater fish (3 species)	28	LD	LD–0.02	Measurable concentration (0.02 mg/kg) in one fish only; limit of detection, 0.005 mg/kg	
1970	Pike (whole body)	10	LD	LD	Limit of detection, 0.005 mg/kg	
1971	Roach (whole body)	6	LD	LD		

Table 5. (contd)

Place and period	Type of sample	No. of samples[a]	Concentration (mg/kg)		Comments	Reference
			Mean	Range[b]		
Wadden Sea (contd)						
1968–69	Hawks and falcons (4 species); liver	16	< 0.1	LD–0.16	Birds found dead or dying; measurable concentration (0.16 mg/kg) in one hawk (buzzard)	Koeman et al. (1969)
	Owls (2 species); liver	3	< 0.1	LD–0.13	Measurable concentration (0.13 mg/kg) in one long-eared owl; limit of detection not specified	
1970	Sandwich tern eggs	10	LD	LD	Limit of detection, 0.02–0.008 mg/kg	Koeman (1971)
1971	Grey heron (*Ardea cinerea*); composite of eggs	27/4	LD	LD		

Table 5. (contd)

Place and period	Type of sample	No. of samples[a]	Concentration (mg/kg)		Comments	Reference
			Mean	Range[b]		
1969–71	Sparrowhawk (*Accipiter nisus*); composite of eggs	28/3	LD	LD		

[a] Sample numbers expressed as n/m correspond to n individuals sampled in m composites analysed
[b] LD, limit of detection

Environmental levels and human exposure

Table 6. Concentrations of endrin in samples collected in North America

Place and period	Type of sample	No. of samples[a]	Concentration (mg/kg)		Comments	Reference
			Mean	Range[b]		
Mississippi River USA						
December 1963	Channel catfish; blood	3	0.44	0.41–0.56	Found dead or dying in areas of extensive fish kills	Anon. (1964)
December 1963	Fish, various species; blood	24	0.18	0.14–0.26		
January–February 1964	Fish, various species; blood	82	0.06	LD–0.21	Caught alive; limit of detection not specified	
July 1964–June 1965	Water	12	<0.01	LD–0.01	4 samples contained measurable concentrations (0.01 mg/kg or litre)	Novak & Rao (1965)
	Mud	12	<0.01	LD–0.01		
	Oysters	12	LD	LD	Limit of detection, 0.005 mg/kg or litre	
	Shrimp	12	LD	LD		
	Fish (2 species)	24	<0.01	LD–0.02	9 samples of fish contained measurable concentrations: 8 of 0.01 mg/kg and 1 of 0.02 mg/kg	

Table 6. (contd)

Place and period	Type of sample	No. of samples[a]	Concentration (mg/kg)		Comments	Reference
			Mean	Range[b]		
Mississippi, USA 1965–72	Eastern oysters (*Crassostrea virginica*); composites of flesh	470	LD	LD	15 or more oysters per composite from 8 sampling stations; limit of detection, 0.01 mg/kg	Butler (1973)
Bayous in the Mississippi delta, USA, October 1968–May 1969	Water	148	LD	LD–0.0002	4 samples contained measurable amounts (0.00009–0.0002 mg/litre); 4 samples contained traces; remainder less than limit of detection	Rowe et al. (1971)
	Sediment	44	LD	LD–0.005	7 samples contained measurable amounts (0.004–0.005 mg/kg); one sample contained a trace	
	Eastern oyster (*Crassostrea virginica*)	111	LD	LD–0.006	79 samples contained < 0.001 mg/kg	

Table 6. (contd)

Place and period	Type of sample	No. of samples[a]	Concentration (mg/kg)		Comments	Reference
			Mean	Range[b]		
Mississippi stream systems 1972–73	Water	26	LD	LD	Samples collected from 13 sampling stations in 5 major river basins; limit of detection, 0.0005 mg/litre	Leard et al. (1980)
	Freshwater bivalves (7 species); flesh	58	LD	LD–0.1	Residues below limit of detection (0.02 mg/kg), except for traces (< 0.1) in 1973 in one river which drains from an agricultural area	
Ontario, 3 streams, 1971	Fish (9 species)		LD	LD	Residues below limit of detection, 0.01 mg/kg	Miles & Harris (1973)
Gulf coast streams, USA	Whole fish (various species); composites	139/48	< 0.02	LD–0.27	Reseidues below limit of detection (0.001 mg/kg) in 33 composites	Henderson et al. (1969)
Mississippi River system, USA		657/202	< 0.01	LD–0.11	Residues in 184 composites below limit of detection (0.001 mg/kg)	

Table 6. (contd)

Place and period	Type of sample	No. of samples[a]	Concentration (mg/kg)		Comments	Reference
			Mean	Range[b]		
Louisiana, USA	Brown pelican (*Pelecanus occidentalis*); eggs				Eggs collected from nests of birds transplanted as nestlings from Florida, 1968–76; limit of detection not specified	Blus et al. (1979)
1971		3	0.10	0.08–0.12		
1972		12	0.18	0.11–0.29		
1973		21	0.16	0.03–0.46		
1974		25	0.30	LD–0.73		
1975		30	0.50	0.29–1.06		
1976		25	0.29	LD–1.47		

[a] Sample numbers expressed as n/m correspond to n individuals sampled in m composites analysed
[b] LD, limit of detection

Environmental levels and human exposure

water (Tarrant & Tatton, 1968), nor in atmospheric air (Abbott et al., 1966); however, endrin has never been used extensively in the United Kingdom.

The mean daily intake of endrin by inhalation in the western part of the Netherlands was calculated on the basis of an air concentration of 41 pg/m^3 (maximum, 300 pg/m^3) to be 0.8 µg/day or 0.3 mg/year, on the basis of air samples taken in the period 1975–81 (Guicherit & Schulting, 1985).

Table 7. Concentrations of endrin in organisms collected in a cotton-growing area in the Republic of Chad in 1969

Sample	No. of samples	Concentration (mg/kg) Mean	Range	Comments
Fish, two species	31	0.02	LD–0.083	Cotton-growing area, endrin and DDT used for pest control; limit of detection, 0.008 mg/kg
Kingfishers and cormorants; liver	46	0.02	LD–0.075	
Birds, non-aquatic, various species				Birds found dead soon after insecticide application; deaths of some birds attributed to endrin
Brain	12	0.51	0.10–0.77	
Liver	12	0.88	0.13–1.42	

From Everaarts et al. (1971); LD, limit of detection

5.1.2 Soil, sediments, and sewage sludge

5.1.2.1 Soil

In the US National Soil Monitoring Program, 1486 soil samples from 37 states were analysed in 1971. Fourteen samples were found to contain endrin, at a geometric mean level of < 0.001 (maximum, 0.02–1.00) mg/kg dry weight (Carey et al., 1978). The mean endrin concentration in 29 soil samples in Kyushu District, Japan, was 0.183 mg/kg (range, 0.016–0.629 mg/kg) dry matter (Suzuki et al., 1973).

5.1.2.2 Sediments

In 1964, levels in the sediment of Cypress Creek, Memphis, TN, USA, upstream and downstream of a pesticide manufacturing plant, reached 12 800 mg/kg dry weight. In 1967, water from the Creek contained levels

Table 8. Concentrations of endrin in organisms collected in a rice-growing area in Wageningen, Surinam

Date	Type of sample	No. of samples[a]	Concentration (mg/kg)		Comments
			Mean	Range[b]	
October 1971	Snail kite (Rostrhamus sociabilis); brain /liver	5/1	LD	LD	Pesticides, including endrin, applied to rice fields
	Black vulture (Coragyps astratus); brain/liver	5/1	LD	LD	
	Egrets (3 species); brain/liver	30/1	LD	LD	Samples collected at end of growing season before insecticide application for next growing season; limit of detection, 0.01 mg/kg
	Purple gallinule (Porphyrula martinica); brain/breast muscle	10/1	LD	LD	
	Spectacled caiman (Caiman crocodilus); brain/liver	10/1	LD	LD	
November 1971	Snail (Pomocea sp.)	10/1	LD	LD	Found dead after application of pentachlorophenol; lower limit of detection, 0.01 mg/kg
	Frog (Pseudis paradoxa); whole-body composites	6/1	LD	LD	
	Kwi kwi (Hoplosternum littorale); whole-body composites	8/1	LD	LD	

Table 8. (contd)

Date	Type of sample	No. of samples[a]	Concentration (mg/kg)[b]		Comments
			Mean	Range	
November 1971 (contd.)					
	Srieba (*Astyanax bimaculatus*); whole-body composites	8/1	LD	0.1	Found dead after application of pentachlorophenol; lower limit of detection 0.01 mg/kg
	Krobia (*Cichlasoma bimaculatum*); whole-body composites	8/1	LD	LD	
	Fish (3 species listed above); whole-body composites	21/3	3.36	1.96–5.35	Found dead after application of endrin
28 November– 4 December 1971	Snail kite; brain	17	LD	LD	Found dead; deaths attributed to pentachlorophenol poisoning
2–9 December 1971	Aquatic birds (4 species); brain	5	0.11	0.06–0.16	Found dead after application of endrin
2–9 December 1971	Wattled jacana (*Jacana jacana*)	1	2.71		Death attributed to endrin poisoning
5–11 December 1971	Common egret (*Egretta alba*); brain	2	0.23	0.14–0.32	Found dead or sick in roost

Table 8. (contd)

Date	Type of sample	No. of samples[a]	Concentration (mg/kg)[b]		Comments
			Mean	Range	
2–11 December 1971	Common egret (*Egretta alba*):				Found dead or sick in rice fields; about half the total endrin was applied during the first half of December
	Brain	9	0.25		
	Liver/kidneys	7–9	0.08		

From Vermeer et al. (1974)
[a] Sample numbers expressed as n/m correspond to n individuals sampled in m composites analysed
[b] LD, limit of detection

Table 9. Concentrations of endrin collected in drainage water from irrigated land, California, USA

Geographical area and year	Type of sample	No. of samples	Concentration (mg/kg or mg/litre) Mean	Range	Comments
Tule Lake and Klamath Lake, National Wildlife Refuge, USA, 1964	Water	44	0.000011	LD–0.0001	Limit of detection, < 0.000003 mg/litre
Refuge, Northern California, USA, April 1965–February 1967	Suspended matter	8	0.011	LD–0.058	
	Vascular plants (two species)	7	0.006	LD–0.013	
	Algae (*Cladophora* sp.)	5	0.007	LD–0.022	Limit of detection, 0.005 mg/kg
	Clam homogenates *Gonidea* sp.)	3	0.013	LD–0.034	
	Fish (*Siphateles* sp.)	5	0.05	0.004–0.198	Samples collected at a pumping station discharging water from irrigated land. Peak concentrations of endrin occurred during the growing season when endrin was applied.

From Godsil & Johnson (1968); LD, limit of detection

Table 10. Concentrations of endrin in environmental samples; residues not associated with particular local use or industrial effluent

Place and period	Type of sample	No. of samples	Concentration (mg/kg)		Comments	Reference
			Mean	Range		
North America						
North Carolina, USA, 1971	Soil (tobacco fields)	19	LD	LD	Limit of detection, 0.01 mg/kg	Reeves et al. (1977)
	Sediment (ponds)	40	LD	LD		
	Frog (*Rana* sp.)	13	LD	LD–0.01		
	Turtle (4 species)	41	LD	LD–0.01		
	Bluegill (*Lepomis macrochirus*)	20	LD	LD		
	Tiger beetle (*Megacephala carolina*)	23	0.02	LD–0.05		
Rice-growing area, Gulf Coast, Texas, USA, 1967–71	Invertebrates, aquatic and terrestrial (various species); whole-body composites of live specimens, except for 4 composites of crayfish	1313/24	LD	LD–trace	A total of 192 dead or dying birds were found in three rice-growing areas in which rice seed dressed with aldrin/ceresan had been used. Endrin residues attributed to use in cotton-growing areas. Limit of detection not defined; trace found in one composite of dead crayfish	Flickinger & King (1972)
1968	Fish (4 species); whole-body composites	542/4	LD	LD		
1968	Cricket frog (*Acris crepeitans blanchardi*); whole-body composites	18/3	LD	LD		

Table 10. (contd)

Place and period	Type of sample	No. of samples	Concentration (mg/kg)		Comments	Reference
			Mean	Range		
1968–70	Turtles (2 species); whole-body composites of live specimens	5/2	LD	LD		
	Snakes (3 species); sick specimens	3	LD	LD		
	Bobcat (sick) and dead rice rat; brain	2	LD	LD		
	Great horned owl; dead specimen; brain	2	LD	LD		
Rice-growing area, Gulf Coast USA, 1967–71	Aquatic birds (10 species) found dead or dying; brain	26	0.22	LD–0.4		
1967	Fulvous tree duck (*Dendrocygna bicolor*); eggs	14	0.1	LD–0.3		
Galveston Bay Texas, USA, 1964	Oyster composites	10	0.01	LD–0.02	Limit of detection, 0.01 mg/kg	Casper (1967)

Table 10. (contd)

Place and period	Type of sample	No. of samples	Concentration (mg/kg)		Comments	Reference
			Mean	Range		
National Monitoring Program: Great Lakes and major river basins, USA (excluding Gulf Coast, Mississippi River system; see Table 6); 1967–68	Fish (various species); whole-body composites	400			93% of samples below limit of detection, 0.001 mg/kg	Henderson et al. (1969)
Atlantic coast streams		741/141	0.002	LD–1.50		
Great Lakes drainage	Fish (various species); whole-body composites	378/66	0.001	LD–0.02		
Hudson Bay, Canada, drainage		51/13	LD	LD		
Colorado River, USA		112/24	0.008	LD–0.71		
Interior basins		120/25	0.001	LD–0.01		
California, USA, streams		90/24	0.002	LD–0.02		
Columbia River, USA, systems		246/64	0.001	LD–0.01		

Table 10. (contd)

Place and period	Type of sample	No. of samples	Concentration (mg/kg)		Comments	Reference
			Mean	Range		
Pacific coast, USA, streams		83/20	LD	LD		
Alaska, USA, streams		105/24	LD	LD		
National Monitoring Program; 50 sampling stations, USA, 1969	Fish (various species); whole-body composites	666/147	LD	LD	Limit of detection, 0.005 mg/kg	Henderson et al. (1971)
Estuaries, California, USA 1966–67	Giant Pacific oyster (*Crassostrea gigas*); Mussel (*Mytilus edulis*); composites of shellfish	1656/138 432/36	0.005 LD	LD–0.01 LD	Measurable concentration in only one oyster; limit of detection, 0.01 mg/kg	Modin (1969)
Arkansas and Mississippi, USA 1970	Catfish from commercial fish farms; composites of edible portions	108–162/54	0.06	LD–0.4	Limit of detection, 0.01 mg/kg; 13 composites contained < 0.01 mg/kg	Crockett et al. (1975)
Intensive cotton-growing areas, Mississippi, USA			0.063	(0.030–0.122)[a]	2 composites contained > 0.3 mg/kg. Significantly higher residues in intensive cotton-growing areas	

Table 10. (contd)

Place and period	Type of sample	No. of samples	Concentration (mg/kg) Mean	Concentration (mg/kg) Range	Comments	Reference
Less intensive cotton-growing areas, Mississippi, USA			0.010	(0.005–0.019)[a]		Crockett et al. (1975)
Major watersheds, USA, 1976	Fish (various species); whole-body composites	582/58	LD	LD	Limit of detection not specified. Intermediate in the manufacture of cyclodiene insecticides detected (mass spectrometry) in Wabash River, Indiana	Veith et al. (1979)
Major watersheds near Great Lakes, USA, 1978	Fish (various species); whole-body composites	138/6	LD	LD	Limit of detection not specified. Endrin identified by mass spectometry in fish from Wabash River, Indiana, together with manufacturing intermediates (concentration not quantified)	Veith et al. (1981)
Arkansas and Mississippi, USA, 1970	Catfish from commercial fish farms, edible portion	50	0.05	LD–0.41	Limit of detection, 0.01 mg/kg; 14 fish contained < 0.01 mg/kg	Hawthorne et al. (1974)

Table 10. (contd)

Place and period	Type of sample	No. of samples	Concentration (mg/kg) Mean	Concentration (mg/kg) Range	Comments	Reference
Continental rise south-east of Cape Hatteras, USA, 1972	Bathyl-demersal fish (*Antimora rostrata*); liver	4	LD	LD	Limit of detection, 0.01 mg/kg. Samples collected by trawling at a depth of 2500 m	Meith-Avcin et al. (1973)
Lake Michigan, USA, 1969–72	Amphipods (*Pontoporeia affinis*) collected from oesophagi of old squaws	24/8	0.08	0.04–0.33	Limit of detection, 0.005 mg/kg	Peterson & Ellarson (1978)
December 1969	Old squaws (*Clangula hyemalis*); carcasses	37	0.18	0.1–0.2	Birds caught in fishing nets or shot	
March–April 1970		44	0.28	0.2–0.4		
December 1970–May 1971		108	0.31	0.1–0.9		
January–February 1972		8	0.6	0.2–1.0		
Northwest Territories and wintering areas other than Lake Michigan, 1971–73		99	0.1	LD–0.3		

Table 10. (contd)

Place and period	Type of sample	No. of samples	Concentration (mg/kg) Mean	Concentration (mg/kg) Range	Comments	Reference
Canada and USA, 1965	Bald eagles (*Haliaeetus leucocephalus*) found dead; brain	29	0.02	LD–0.1	Limit of detection, 0.05 mg/kg. Concentration in 24 specimens below limit of detection	Reichel et al. (1969)
Connecticut & Florida, USA, 1967–68	Bald eagles found dead; brain, liver, carcass	2	LD	LD–0.1	Limit of detection not defined; apparent concentration of 0.1 mg/kg in Florida eagle not confirmed by thin-layer chromatography	Reichel et al. (1969)
Continental USA 1966 1967 1968	Bald eagle: brain	21 21 26	LD LD LD	LD LD LD	Limit of detection, 0.05 mg/kg	Mulhern et al. (1970)
1969 1970	Bald eagle: brain	28 11	LD LD	LD LD	Limit of detection, 0.05 mg/kg	Belisle et al. (1972)
1971–72	Bald eagle: brain	37	LD	LD	Limit of detection, 0.05 mg/kg	Cromartie et al. (1975)

Table 10. (contd)

Place and period	Type of sample	No. of samples	Concentration (mg/kg)		Comments	Reference
			Mean	Range		
Continental USA (contd)						
1973–74	Bald eagle; brain	81	LD	LD	Limit of detection, 0.05 mg/kg	Prouty et al. (1977)
1975	Bald eagle; brain	49	0.07	LD–0.50	Limit of detection, 0.05 mg/kg. Concentrations in 46 specimens < 0.05 mg/kg	Kaiser et al. (1980)
1976		50	0.08	LD–0.71	Concentrations in 44 specimens below limit of detection. Death of one eagle attributed to endrin poisong	
1977		69	0.08	LD–1.2	Concentrations in 64 specimens below limit of detection. Death of one eagle attributed to endrin poisoning	
Wisconsin, Maine, Florida, USA, 1968	Bald eagle; eggs	26	LD	LD	Limit of detection, 0.05 mg/kg	Krantz et al. (1970)

Table 10. (contd)

Place and period	Type of sample	No. of samples	Concentration (mg/kg) Mean	Concentration (mg/kg) Range	Comments	Reference
USA, 1964–71	Golden eagle (*Aquila chrysaetos*) found dead or dying; body fat	102	LD	LD–0.3	Limit of detection, 0.1 mg/kg. Concentrations in 97 specimens below limit of detection	Reidinger & Crabtree (1974)
Coast of California, USA, 1968–69	Gray whale (*Eschrichtius robustus*); blubber	23	LD	LD		Wolman & Wilson (1970)
	Sperm whale (*Physeter catodon*); blubber	6	LD	LD		
South Atlantic and Pacific Oceans, 1968–69	Small cetaceans (10 species); blubber, brain, muscle	69	LD	LD–0.24	Limit of detection, 0.1 mg/kg. Measurable concentrations (0.22 and 0.24 mg/kg) found in two specimens	O'Shea et al. (1980)
Maryland, USA, 1976	Little brown bat (*Myotis lucifugus*); carcass	87	LD	LD	Limit of detection, 0.1 mg/kg	Clark & Krynitsky (1978)
Missouri, USA 1976–77	Gray bat (*Myotis grisescens*) found dead; carcass (lipid basis)	20	LD	LD	Limit of detection, 0.1 mg/kg	Clark et al. (1980)

Table 10. (contd)

Place and period	Type of sample	No. of samples	Concentration (mg/kg) Mean	Concentration (mg/kg) Range	Comments	Reference
Washington Sate (orchards), October 1981–July 1982	18 bird species (total number of birds, 91) Brain Eggs	78 53		LD–> 0.8 LD–1.7		Blus et al. (1983)
Detroit River, Niagara River, Saginaw Bay, USA, 1978–82	Herring gulls (*Larus argentatus*); eggs		LD	LD		Struger et al. (1985)
North-west Atlantic Ocean, Gulf of Mexico, USA, 1973–75	Fish species; muscle	700	0.008	LD–0.026		Stout (1980)
South-east Montana, USA, 1978–81	Merlins (*Falco columbarius*); eggs		LD	LD		Becker & Sieg (1987)
New Jersey, Maryland, USA	Snapping turtles (*Chelydra serpentina*)	11	LD	LD	Limit of detection, 0.1 mg/kg	Albers et al. (1986)
Florida, USA	Snail kite (*Rostrhamus sociabilis*); eggs, nestlings		LD	LD	Limit of detection, 0.05 mg/kg	Sykes (1985)

Table 10. (contd)

Place and period	Type of sample	No. of samples	Concentration (mg/kg) Mean	Range	Comments	Reference
Missouri, USA, 1982	Gray bats (*Myotis grisescens*)	7	LD	LD		Clawson & Clark (1989)
	Red bats (*Lasiurus borealis*)	7	LD	LD		
	Pipstrelles (*Pipistrellus subflavus*)	2	LD	LD		
Denver, Colorado, USA, 1980–81	Tree swallows (*Tachycineta bicolor*)	32	LD	LD		Deweese et al. (1985)
North-east Alberta, Canada, 1980–82	Otter (*Lutra canadensis*); carcass	158	LD	LD	Limit of detection, 0.001 mg/kg	Somers et al. (1987)
Africa						
Lake Nakuru, Kenya, 1970	Fish (*Tilapia graham*); whole-body composites	10–20/2	LD	LD	Limit of detection: fish, 0.002 mg/kg; birds, 0.009 mg/kg	Koeman & Santiago (1972)
	African cormorant (*Phalacrocorax africanus*) liver	3	LD	LD		
	White pelican (*Pelicanus onocratalus*)	1	LD	LD		
	Lesser flamingo (*Phoeniconaias minor*)	5	LD	LD		

Table 10. (contd)

Place and period	Type of sample	No. of samples	Concentration (mg/kg) Mean	Concentration (mg/kg) Range	Comments	Reference
Europe						
Province of Leon, Spain, 1986	Kestrels (*Falco tinnunculus*); 5 organs or tissues	4	—	LD–2.0	Liver, 0.01; brain, 0.016; kidneys, 0.027; muscle, 0.054 mg/kg	Sierra & Santiago (1987)
	Sparrowhawk (*Accipiter nisus*)	3		LD–2.0	Liver, 0.139; kidneys, 0.4; fat, 1.068; brain, 0.031; muscle, 0.047 mg/kg	
	Red kite (*Milvus milvus*)	2		LD–2.0	Kidneys, 0.005; brain, 0.103; fat, 2.035 mg/kg	
1984–87	Barn owl (*Tyto alba*)			0.001–0.22	Liver, 0.036; brain, 0.052; kidneys, 0.034; fat, 0.014; muscle, 0.020 mg/kg	Sierra et al. (1987)
North Sea	*Gadus morhua* and *Merlangius merlangus*; ovary	12 4		0.0001–0.0023 < 0.001–0.0011		Von Westernhagen et al. (1987)
North Sea	*Merlangius merlangus* Ovary Testis Liver	56 16 30		LD–0.001 LD LD		Von Westernhagen et al. (1989)

Sample numbers expressed as n/m correspond to n individuals sampled in m composites analysed; LD, limit of detection
[a] 95% confidence interval

of 0.27-2.03 µg/litre and sediment contained levels of 47.4–10 676 mg/kg dry weight (Barthel et al., 1969).

Endrin was found in 17% of samples of bottom sediment from 59 sites on the Detroit River, USA, at levels up to 43 µg/kg (limit of detection, 1.0 µg/kg) (Hamdy & Post, 1985). No endrin was detected in sediment samples collected in 1980–82 from riverine and pothole wetlands at 17 locations in the north–central USA (Martin & Hartman, 1985) or in samples of sediment from 34 stations on the upper Great Lakes in 1974 (< 1 µg/kg) (Glooschenko et al., 1976).

None of 60 samples of bottom deposit collected in 1974 from 19 rivers and their estuaries in Japan contained endrin (< 0.01 mg/kg) (Japanese Environmental Agency, 1975).

No endrin was detected in sediment and particulates from the River Elbe in Germany in 1983–85 (Sturm et al., 1986). Sediment from Rotterdam Harbour contained a total of 3–59 µg/kg aldrin, dieldrin, and endrin. No endrin was found at seven sites in the Elbe Estuary (Japenga et al., 1987). A housing estate in the Netherlands, comprising about 800 houses and public buildings, was built in 1983 directly on a 4-m-thick layer of harbour sludge transferred in 1962–64 from about 20 harbour basins in Rotterdam and the industrial area around the Nieuwe Waterweg. Organic solvents, polycyclic aromatic hydrocarbons, heavy metals, and endrin and related pesticides, were detected in the sludge. One-third of the soil samples collected in the gardens (71 locations), 0–40 cm below the surface, contained endrin and related pesticides at a mean concentration of 1.2 mg/kg and a maximal concentration of 19.5 mg/kg dry weight (Van Wynen & Stijkel, 1988).

In surface sediments from five sites in Manukan Harbour, New Zealand, only traces (none detected to < 0.1 µg/kg dry weight) of endrin were found (Fox et al., 1988).

Particulates from two sites in the Shatt al Arab River in Iraq contained endrin at 84 and 154 µg/kg, and a site in the Tigris River contained 217 µg/kg. No endrin was found in the Euphrates River. The mean concentration of endrin in surface and subsurface sediment from the Shatt al Arab River ranged from 3 to 18 (range, none detected to 32) µg/kg; no endrin was found in surface and subsurface sediment from the Tigris River. None was found in surface sediment from the Euphrates River, but in subsurface

Environmental levels and human exposure

sediment a mean concentration of 11 (5–25) μg/kg was detected (DouAbul et al., 1988).

5.1.2.3 Sewage sludge

Endrin was found in only a few of 444 sludge samples analysed from sewage treatment works in the United Kingdom. The mean concentration was 0.11 mg/kg of sludge, with a range of 0.01–0.71 mg/kg (McIntyre & Lester, 1984). All samples of non-disinfected influent at a pilot plant in Jefferson Parish, LA, USA, contained endrin, at an average concentration of 0.67 (0.25–1.58) ng/litre (Lykins et al., 1986).

Sludge from three main waste water treatment plants in Kuwait was analysed over a 6-month period in 1984-85. Two grab samples were taken from each plant every month to give a total of 36 samples. The mean endrin levels for the three plants were 0.02, 0.02, and 0.06 mg/kg (Samhan & Ghobrial, 1987). Sewage plant effluents before and after treatment were analysed in Baghdad (Iraq) in 1982–83. Endrin was found in 8/15 samples taken before treatment, at a mean concentration of 0.291 (0.081–2.637) μg/litre, and in 6/15 samples taken after treatment, at a mean concentration of 0.194 (0.072–1.197) μg/litre (Al-Omar et al., 1985a).

5.1.3 Water

5.1.3.1 Surface water

Data on the concentrations of endrin in surface water concern mainly those regions in the USA where use of endrin was widespread, such as in Mississippi and Missouri, over the period 1957–65. The highest concentrations were found in 1963 in the Lower Mississippi, with a maximum level of 0.214 μg/litre. The concentrations and the rate of occurrence decreased considerably later (Breidenbach et al., 1967). In a survey in 1964–68, a maximal level of 0.133 μg/litre was reported to have been found in the Missouri basin in 1967. No endrin was detected in 1968 (Lichtenberg et al., 1970). In 1974, the concentrations in the Lower Mississippi was 0.0045 μg/litre in August–November (Brodtmann, 1976).

In one sample from the Potomac River, at Quantico, endrin and endrin aldehyde were identified at concentrations of 0.005 and 0.006 μg/litre, respectively (Hall et al., 1987). Endrin was not found in the waters near the Los Angeles County ocean outfalls (< 0.00005 μg/litre) (Green et al.,

1986) or in surface water in Louisiana in 1980 (< 1.0 ng/litre) (McFall et al., 1985). In a programme to monitor surface water in the USA in 1976–80, endrin was found in only 0.1% of samples, at a maximum value of 0.04 µg/litre (Carey & Kutz, 1985).

No endrin was found in water from 33 sites in the Upper Great Lakes in Canada (< 0.01 µg/litre) (Glooschenko et al., 1976). In Ontario, where endrin was used only sparingly, no residues were found in 1971 or 1975–77 (Miles & Harris, 1973; Frank et al., 1981). In water samples taken 1 m below the surface at 14 stations on Lake Ontario in 1983, endrin was found in concentrations of 0.000044–0.000145 µg/litre (Biberhofer & Stevens, 1987).

In a survey of the aquatic environment in The Netherlands, including drinking-water, 1826 samples were taken at 99 sampling sites between September 1969 and 1977; traces of endrin were reported occasionally (Wegman & Greve, 1978, 1980). Studies of surface water in other areas in Europe failed to show the presence of endrin (Wilson Committee, 1969; Engst & Knoll, 1973; Uhnak et al., 1974; Galassi & Provini, 1981; Hrubec, 1988). In 1984–85, water from a number of rivers in Germany contained endrin at levels of none detected to 0.30 µg/litre (Braun ,1985); surface water in Greece occasionally contained levels of 0.0003–0.0004 µg/litre (Albanis et al., 1986).

No endrin was found in surface or drinking-water in the state of Saõ Paulo (Brazil) (Lara & Barreto, 1972), but it was found in water reservoirs of basins in Saõ Paulo at concentrations of none detected to 1.02 µg/litre (Celeste & Caceres, 1987; Caceres et al., 1987). Endrin was also found accidentally in two lagoons in north-west Mexico (Rosales et al., 1985).

None of 60 water samples collected in 1974 from 19 rivers and their estuaries in Japan contained endrin (< 0.1 µg/litre) (Japanese Environmental Agency, 1975).

Endrin was found at five places in the River Nile at concentrations of 0.0038–0.0189 µg/litre in March–September 1982 (El-Dib & Badawy, 1985). In analyses of the water of the Shatt al Arab, Euphrates, and Tigris Rivers, endrin was found only in the Euphrates River, but in all samples at a mean concentration of 0.024 (0.014–0.036) µg/litre (DouAbul et al., 1988). It occurred in 75% of samples of urban, industrial, and continental water from the Moroccan Mediterranean coast, at concentrations of none

Environmental levels and human exposure

detected to 13 µg/litre (Kassabi et al., 1988). Three of 15 grab samples of surface water sources in Southern Africa (Orange Free State) contained endrin, at a concentration of 2–4 µg/litre (Hassett et al., 1987).

Endrin was present in the Kalinadi River in India as a result of runoff, especially from agricultural areas, at a concentration of 2 µg/litre (Kudesia & Bali, 1985). In the Chao Phraya River and klongs in Bangkok, Thailand, no endrin (< 0.001 µg/litre) was found in 1984 (Onodera & Tabucanon, 1986). Analyses in Bali of 16 samples of river water in the dry season and 15 samples in the rainy season showed the presence of endrin at 40 µg/litre once, in the rainy season (Machbub et al., 1988).

5.1.3.2 Rain and snow

No endrin was found (limit of detection, 1–2 ng/litre) in atmospheric precipitation in the form of snow (17 samples in 1976) and rain (81 samples in 1976 and 1977) on the Canadian side of the Great Lakes and inland in areas remote from any nearby industrial or urban contamination (Strachan et al., 1980). Four of 16 samples of rain-water collected at four sites in Canada had levels of 0.00013–0.00044 µg/litre and another sample had 0.0048 µg/litre; no endrin was detected in the other 11 samples. The mean endrin contents in samples taken at another site in 1977, 1981, 1983, and 1984 were none detected, 0.000065, 0.000085, and 0.000049 µg/litre, respectively (Strachan, 1988). Endrin was not detected in snow samples collected at 12 sites in the Northwest Territories of Canada in 1985–86 (Gregor & Gummer, 1989).

5.1.3.3 Drinking-water

Data obtained in 1964–67 from selected municipal drinking-water treatment plants in Mississippi and Missouri, USA, showed that the concentration in approximately 10% of the samples exceeded 0.1 µg/litre in the first year but that the concentrations were lower in 1965–67 (Schafer et al., 1969). The most recent study on US drinking-water was done on finished water in New Orleans, LA, in 1974, where the highest concentration measured was 4 ng/litre (US EPA, 1974).

During 1976, endrin was found at a mean concentration of 4 ng/litre (range, 1–7 ng/litre) in drinking-water in Ottawa, Canada (Williams et al., 1978).

The mean concentration of endrin in drinking-water at the El-Abbasia station, Egypt, in 1986 was 3.507 ± 1.45 ng/litre in 10 samples taken before purification and 1.845 ± 1.29 ng/litre after purification (Abdel-Razik et al., 1988).

Drinking-water from the North Coast region of New South Wales, Australia, was analysed in 1986–87: 147 of 659 samples contained traces of endrin (none detected [< 0.005] to 0.05 µg/litre) (Ang et al., 1989).

5.1.3.4 Groundwater

Water in wells used as a source of water for mixing pesticides in fruit orchards in West Virginia (USA) was found to contain endrin at about 1 ng/litre in 1985 and in 1986. The water in these wells was not used for drinking-water. Endrin had not been used in the area since 1970, and the authors cite their results as evidence for the persistence of endrin and its capacity to contaminate groundwater many years after cessation of use (Hogmire et al., 1990).

5.1.4 Organisms in the environment

5.1.4.1 Birds

Endrin was found in the carcasses of four of 16 turkey vultures (*Cathartes aura*) in southern California, USA, in 1981, at levels of 0.11–0.23 mg/kg wet weight, but in none of six common ravens (*Corvus corax*). It was also found in two of four vulture eggs, at 0.10 (range, none detected to 0.52) mg/kg wet weight, but in none of 30 raven eggs (Wiemeyer et al., 1986).

Endrin was found in eggs of shag (*Phalacrocorax aristotelis*) and cormorants (*Phalacrocorax carbo*) at one of five collection sites in the east, south-east, and south of Ireland, at a geometric mean concentration of 0.30 (range, 0.06–1.60) µg/kg (Wilson & Earley, 1986). Eggs from two species of passerine birds, three species of gull, four species of tern, and the night heron were collected in Italy in 1982–83. Endrin was found in 30 eggs of the night heron (*Nicticorax nycticorax*), at an average concentration of 0.11 (0.03–0.27) mg/kg, in 50 eggs of the gull-billed tern (*Gelochelidon nilotica*), at a concentration of 0.28 (0.05–1.31) mg/kg, and in 38 eggs of the tree sparrow (*Passer montanus*) and 33 eggs of the hooded crow (*Corvus corone*), at concentrations of 0.17 (0.09–0.33) and 0.21 (0.07–

0.31) mg/kg. It was not detected in eggs of the other species (Fasola et al., 1987).

No endrin was found in 98 eggs or in the livers of 112 nestlings of rooks (*Corvus frugilegus*) collected from five rookeries in northern Germany in 1982–83 (Beyerbach et al., 1987) or in 45 eggs and the livers of eight young lapwings (*Vanellus vanellus*) collected in 1984 and 1986 (Beyerbach et al., 1988).

Detectable residues of the commonest organochlorine pesticides were found in 0.9% of 112 pools (mostly of 10 birds) of starlings (*Sturnus vulgaris*) collected in 129 sites in the USA in 1979 and in 1.6% of 129 pools in 1982. In most states, no endrin was detected, but levels of 0.01 and 0.17 mg/kg wet weight were found in two (Bunck et al., 1987).

Endrin was present at microgram levels per kilogram of wet weight in 272 samples of liver, muscle, fat, and eggs from northern fulmars (*Fulmarus glacialis*), black-legged kittiwakes (*Rissa tridactyla*), and thick-billed murres (*Uria lomvia*) collected in 1975–77 on Prince Leopold Island, Northwest Territories, Canada (Nettleship & Peakall, 1987). It was found in 8 of 108 carcasses of herons analysed in the USA since 1966, at levels of 0.10–0.86 mg/kg wet weight (Ohlendorf et al., 1981) but was not found in 255 pools of wings from black ducks (*Anas rubripes*) and mallards (*A. platyrhynchos*) collected in the USA in 1981–82 (Prouty & Bunck, 1986).

Endrin was not detected in six eggs of Forster's tern (*Sterna forsteri*) collected on Green Bay and Lake Poygan, Michigan, USA in 1983 (Kubiak et al., 1989). None was found in a total of 107 eggs collected in 1975–80 from 10 species of colonial waterbirds nesting in areas around Green Bay and Lake Michigan. The species were little gulls (*Lares minutes*), green-backed herons (*Butorides striatus*), black terns (*Chlidonias niger*), herring gulls (*L. argentatus*), ring-billed gulls (*L. delawarensis*), common terns (*S. hirundo*), Forster's tern (*S. forsteri*), double-crested cormorants (*Phalcrocorax auritis*), black-crowned night herons (*Nycticorax nycticorax*), and cattle egrets (*Bubulcus ibis*). The limit of detection was 0.1 mg/kg in 1977 and 0.05 mg/kg in 1978 (Heinz et al., 1985).

Of five eggs from peregrine falcons (*Falco peregrinus*) collected in Arizona, USA, in 1978–82, one collected in 1978 contained endrin at 0.20 mg/kg dry weight, one collected in 1981 contained no detectable amount (< 0.01 mg/kg) and three collected in 1982 contained 0.02–0.04 mg/kg (Ellis et al., 1989).

No endrin was detected in 27 eggs from tree sparrows (*Passer montanus*), 4 eggs from house martins (*Delichon urbica*), 28 eggs from white storks (*Ciconia ciconia*), or eggs from nine other species of bird in Germany in 1984. The livers of 25 nestling, 13 young, and 17 adult white storks also contained no detectable level of this pesticide (limit of detection, 0.001 mg/kg) (Heidmann et al., 1989).

5.1.4.2 Fish and shellfish

The endrin concentrations in red mullet (*Mullet barbatus*) collected at six locations in the Pagassitikos Gulf (Greece) in 1986–87 were < 0.005–0.5 µg/kg fresh weight of fillets (Satsmadjis et al., 1988). The mean concentrations in liver, brain, kidneys, and muscle of 22 trout (*Salmo trutta fario* L.) taken from four rivers in Leon, Spain, in 1985 were 0.104, 0.123, 0.157, and 0.157 mg/kg wet weight. The incidence in the four organs was 4.54–22.73% (Teran & Sierra, 1987). Endrin was found in 29 samples of fish collected in Italy, at a median concentration of 0.019 mg/kg (Cantoni et al., 1988). Organochlorine compounds were measured in three samples of liver from cod (*Gadus morhua*) collected in three areas of the North Sea in 1977–87; endrin was present at a concentration of < 5 µg/kg of product (De Boer, 1989).

Endrin was not detected (< 0.01 mg/kg) in two or three replicate samples, each comprising three to five bluegill (*Lepomis macrochirus*) and common carp (*Cyprinus carpio*), collected from downstream sites exposed to irrigated agriculture and from non-irrigated upstream sites on the San Joaquin River and tributaries in California, USA (Saiki & Schmitt, 1986). Endrin was also not found in water near Los Angeles County ocean outfalls (< 0.00005 µg/litre) or in mussels (*Mytilus californianus*) (< 0.1 µg/kg wet weight) that had been suspended at the monitoring site for 2 months to provide a measure of the bioaccumulation of chlorinated hydrocarbon contaminants (Green et al., 1986). No endrin was detected in fish samples taken at nine locations in north–central USA (Martin & Hartman, 1985), and endrin was not detectable (< 0.001 mg/kg) in 527 samples of edible fin fish harvested from Chesapeake Bay and its tributaries (Maryland) over the period 1976–80 or in 20 samples of roe and gonadal tissue (Eisenberg & Topping, 1985).

No detectable quantity (< 1 µg/kg) of endrin was found in two species of crayfish (*Procambarus clarkii* and *P. acutus*) commercially harvested from dual-cropped ponds and from waters of the Atchafalaya River Basin and the Mississippi River in southern Louisiana, or in sediment and water collected from several ponds and at the Basin three times during 1986 and 1987 (Madden et al., 1989).

Endrin was measured at levels of 0.4 and 66 µg/kg in American eels (*Anguilla rostrata*) sampled at various sites between Lake Ontario and the mouth of the St Lawrence river in 1982 (Castonguay et al., 1989). Endrin was not detectable (< 0.002 mg/kg) in 'most' composite samples (1–15 fish of 10 different species) collected from 10 sites on the Great Lakes and tributaries between 1980 and 1981, although in a few cases concentrations up to 0.01 mg/kg were found (Devault, 1985). Endrin was not present (< 0.005 mg/kg) in fillets of Fall Run Coho salmon (*Oncorhynchus kisutch*) taken from 14 sites on the Great Lakes in 1984. In most cases, three samples per site were analysed, and the fish were 2–3 years old (Devault et al., 1988). Johnson et al. (1988) measured the input of organochlorine pesticides from precipitation and runoff to five small lakes peripheral to the Canadian Great Lakes and the levels of residues in fish caught in the lakes. While endrin was detectable in precipitation (at 0.46 and 0.54 ng/litre at the two sampling sites), none was measured in runoff water and no detectable residue was found in fish.

The mean concentrations of endrin in 13 commercially important fish species collected in the north-west Arabian Gulf varied between 1 and 28 µg/kg, and those in five species collected from Hor al-Hammar Lake in Iraq in 1985 were 3–67 µg/kg wet weight of edible tissue. Endrin residues were detected in approximately 90% of the fish (DouAbul et al., 1987a). Samples of *Barbus xanthopetrus* collected in the Shatt al Arab River and in Hor al Hammar Lake contained average concentrations of 4 (none detected to 9) and 20 (11–27) µg/kg, while Indian shed (*Tenualosa ilistra*) from the Shatt al Arab River contained 80 (57–108) µg/kg (wet weight). Shrimp (*Metapanaeus affinis*) did not contain endrin (DouAbul et al., 1987b). In 1984, *B. xanthopetrus* from the River contained a mean concentration of 16 µg/kg wet weight, and those from the Lake, 154 µg/kg (range, 13–355); Indian shed had mean concentrations of 41–147 µg/kg (range, none detected to 236) (DouAbul et al., 1987c). Freshwater mussel (*Corbicula fluminea*) collected in the Shatt al Arab River contained 166–540 µg/kg (range, 140–583) (DouAbul et al., 1988). Endrin was present at concentrations of 1.9–12.2 µg/kg of muscle tissue (wet weight) in three fish species and at 0.88–7.7 µg/kg in three *Tilapia* species collected near Alexandria, Egypt, in 1985 (El Nabawi et al., 1987).

Endrin was present at 0.003–0.004 mg/kg in black pomfret (*Parastromateus niger*), mackerel (*Rastrelliger kanagurta*), and marine vala (*Chirocentrus* sp.) and at 0.08 mg/kg in tuna (*Euthynnus affinis*) collected off the Indian coast (Radhakrishnan & Antony, 1989). It was found in one sample of fish at 0.019 mg/kg wet weight and in one shellfish sample at 0.034 mg/kg but in none of 312 other specimens of 11 types of fish, crustaceans, and molluscs obtained from five sites in Java, Indonesia (limit of detection, 0.01 mg/kg) (Koeman et al., 1974).

No endrin was found (< 0.005 mg/kg) in 60 samples of fish and shellfish collected in 19 rivers and their estuaries in Japan in 1974 (Japanese Environmental Agency, 1975).

The median concentration of endrin in the eggs of 15 adult chinook salmon (*Onchorhynchus tshawytscha*) collected in Lake Michigan in 1982 was 23.5 µg/kg wet weight (range, 3.9-126.3) (Giesy et al., 1986).

Composite samples of whole fish of selected species were collected in 1983 near the shores of 13 tributaries of Lake Michigan and Grand Traverse Bay. Two of each of the following species were collected from each site: common carp (*Cyprinus carpio*), bowfin (*Amia calva*), channel catfish (*Ictalurus punctatus*), pumpkinseed (*Lepomis gibbosus*), rock bass (*Ambloplites rupestris*), small-mouth bass (*Micropterus dolomieui*), large-mouth bass (*M. salmoides*), lake trout (*Salvelinus namaycush*), and pike (*Esox lucius*); the composites comprised 3–11 fish. Endrin was not detected (limit, 0.005 mg/kg) (Camanzo et al., 1987).

Yellow perch (*Perca flavencens*) were sampled in eight reservoirs and lakes in Ohio and Wisconsin, USA, in 1978–79. Endrin was found in four fish at levels of 0.008–0.02 mg/kg, which were much lower than the levels found of polychlorinated biphenyls, DDT and dieldrin (Carline & Lawal, 1985).

5.1.4.3 Mixed species

Herons (*Nyctanassa violacea*), water snakes (*Natrix* spp.), raccoons (*Procyon lotor*), channel catfish (*Ictalurus punctatus*), crappies (*Pomoxis* spp.), frogs (*Rana* spp.), and crawfish (*Procambarus clarkii*) were collected from three watersheds in Louisiana, USA in 1978–79. Endrin was found in a heron at 0.014 mg/kg and in a catfish at 0.022 mg/kg, but in no other case (limit of detection, < 0.05 mg/kg) (Dowd et al., 1985).

Environmental levels and human exposure

5.1.5 Other food and feed

5.1.5.1 Cereals

Endrin has been used extensively for the control of insect pests in rice. Typically, one to four applications are made, depending on local conditions, the last application usually not later than one month before harvest. Data on residue levels are available from India (1969–70), Thailand (1968–70), the Philippines, Indonesia (1966), and Venezuela (1969). The levels in polished rice were 0.01–0.04 mg/kg of product (mean, 0.014 mg/kg), except in India where higher levels in the order of 0.12 mg/kg were found. Bran, which is used mainly as a component of poultry feed, contained a mean level of 0.35 mg/kg (range, < 0.01–2.3 mg/kg), and low levels of delta-ketoendrin were found (FAO/WHO, 1971).

Endrin has been used to only a limited extent on grain crops. The residues in different types of treated grains in the USA were generally below 0.05 mg/kg of product, except in oats in which levels up to 0.5 mg/kg were found. In India, up to five applications on sorghum gave residue levels below 0.02 mg/kg; in the USA, the levels in sorghum were below 0.05 mg/kg. Straw of cereals contains higher levels: rice straw had up to 3 mg/kg,, and sorghum straw up to 0.4 mg/kg (FAO/WHO, 1971).

Wheat imported into the United Kingdom in 1987–88 did not contain endrin (< 0.01 mg/kg) (Osborne et al., 1989).

5.1.5.2 Fruit and vegetables

Endrin is occasionally used for control of field mice (voles). No residue was found in apples at harvest (detection limit, 0.01–0.002 mg/kg of whole fruit) when it was sprayed on the ground under trees in orchards in autumn or spring. The levels were sometimes higher in fallen fruit, ranging from < 0.002 to 0.02 mg/kg of product (Horsfall et al., 1970; FAO/WHO, 1971).

Only 14 of 15 000 samples of fruit and vegetables imported into Sweden during the period 1981–84 contained endrin, at a maximum concentration of 0.02 mg/kg (Anderson, 1986). The pesticide analysis programme of the Swedish National Food Administration on fruit and vegetables, including potatoes, showed no residue of endrin above the limit of detection of 0.02 mg/kg in 13 724 samples analysed in 1985–87 (B.G. Ericsson, personal communication, 1990). The mean endrin concentration in 137 samples of grape products (including seeds, skins, marc and lees) in Italy was 6.2–16.2 µg/kg (Marinelli et al., 1986). Seven of 306 samples of apples (five types) collected in 1980–83 from five regions of Italy contained endrin (limit of detection, 0.001 mg/kg) (Foschi et al., 1985).

In Pakistan, in 16 samples of cucumber sprayed at the time of maturity with a 0.05% endrin solution at a rate of 100 gallons/acre (1123 litres/ha), the endrin concentrations ranged from 3.04 to 6.69 mg/kg. The residues persisted in the edible portion of cucumber up to 14 days and diminished thereafter (Illahi et al., 1986). Endrin was found in 17% of samples of peas collected from fields and markets in Faisalabad, Pakistan, at a level of 1.3–4.32 µg/kg. The residues persisted for up to 12 days and then decreased (Illahi et al., 1987). No endrin was found (< 0.02 mg/kg) in 141 samples of fruit and vegetables from Pakistan in 1982–83 (Masud & Farhat, 1985).

In an analysis of soya bean and soya bean straw in a US monitoring programme, seven of 177 samples of soya beans contained a geometrical mean of < 0.001 (maximum, 0.03) mg/kg, and one of eight straw samples contained < 0.01 mg/kg (Carey et al., 1978). Endrin was used in up to four applications on sugar-cane in the USA, with an interval of 45 days or longer between the last application and harvest. The residues found in cane were usually < 0.05 mg/kg of product (FAO/WHO, 1971).

5.1.5.3 Meat, poultry, and chicken eggs

Bovine fat (40 samples), pig fat (45 samples), calf fat (45 samples), sheep fat (22 samples), poultry fat (42 samples), and eggs (44 samples) analysed in the Netherlands in 1983 had a median endrin concentration of < 0.04 mg/kg (Dutch Agricultural Advisory Commission on Environmental Pollutants, 1983). No endrin was found (detection limit, 0.005 mg/kg) in samples of beef, pork, goat, mutton, poultry, or eggs analaysed in Italy in 1985–87 (Cantoni et al., 1988) or in 'most' samples of pork, rabbit, or poultry analysed in Rheinland/Pfalz, Germany, in 1981–84 (Kampe, 1985). Dietary surveys in the United Kingdom demonstrated no endrin in meat (detection limit, 0.02 mg/kg) (United Kingdom Ministry of Agriculture, Fisheries and Food, 1989).

Endrin was present in 10.8% of 2032 samples of bovine fat from carcasses collected from slaughterhouses in Brazil, at a mean level of

Environmental levels and human exposure

0.01 mg/kg; the highest level was 0.09 mg/kg of tissue (De Paula Carvalho et al., 1984). Endrin was present in hens' eggs from four of five areas in Mexico, at concentrations of 0.004–0.11 mg/kg of whole egg, and in 11 of 16 samples of chicken meat, at an average concentration of 0.12 (none detected to 0.6) mg/kg on a fat basis (Albert, 1990).

Endrin was detected in 86 of 221 samples of hens' eggs (78 native and 143 commercial) collected in 1975–77 in Iran, at a mean concentration of 0.017 (range, 0.003–0.13) mg/kg (Hashemy-Tonkabony & Mosstofian, 1979). No endrin was found (limit of detection, 0.02 mg/kg) in samples of about 25 eggs of *sawah* ducks collected on 11 local markets in Java, Indonesia, in 1972 (Koeman et al., 1974).

It was found in 14 of 367 hens' eggs collected from 61 farms in 11 districts of Kenya in 1984; in three of the eggs, the level was > 0.2 mg/kg (Mugambi et al., 1989).

Heating, baking, frying, and steaming of tissues obtained from broilers fed endrin at 10 mg/kg of diet for 8 weeks did not significantly reduce the level of residues: raw, 28.2; baked, 20.8; fried, 22.7; and steamed, 19.4 mg/kg of dry tissue (Ritchey et al., 1972).

5.1.5.4 Milk and milk products

The mean endrin concentration in 20 samples of fresh buffalo milk in Kalubia, Egypt, was 0.02 mg/kg of milk fat (range, < 0.01–0.03 mg/kg (Abdou et al., 1983). Cows' milk (39 samples) collected in four areas of Bagdad, Iraq, in 1981–82 contained a mean of 60 (none detected to 400) µg/litre (Al-Omar et al., 1985b).

The average concentration of endrin in 10 samples of evaporated cows' milk from three main cities in the agricultural region of Mexico was < 0.007 mg/litre of milk fat (Albert et al.,1982). Endrin was found in powdered milk at an average concentration of 0.06 mg/kg and in cheese at a concentration of 10–27.2 mg/kg on a fat basis (Albert, 1990).

The level of endrin in milk in the USA was < 0.001 mg/litre (on a fat basis) (FAO/WHO, 1971). No endrin (< 0.5 µg/litre) was found in 308 samples from bulk transports of milk collected in Ontario, Canada, in 1977 (Frank et al., 1979) or in 359 samples collected in 1983 (Frank et al., 1985).

No residue was found (detection limit, < 0.005 mg/kg) in samples of milk, cream, butter, and cheese in Italy (Cantoni et al., 1988) or in 12 samples of cows' milk collected in 1984–86 from different areas of Spain (< 0.01 mg/kg fat) (Barcelo & Puignou, 1987).

5.1.5.5 Fat and oils

The most important use of endrin is for the control of insects in cotton, the number of applications being 1–12; cottonseed oil is used for cooking and for the manufacture of margarine, while the extracted cake is used as cattle feed. Endrin is thus present both in the cottonseed and in the edible oil and cakes. In a study of the extraction processes, it was found that alkali washing and bleaching had no marked effect but that deodorization reduced the endrin levels to below the limit of detection (0.03 mg/kg) (Smith et al., 1968).

In field studies carried out in the USA, cottonseed contained endrin at a maximum of 0.1 mg/kg, although the levels were usually much lower. delta-Ketoendrin was not detected. The levels in crude, decolourized, and deodorized oil in Venezuela and Brazil were all < 0.02 mg/kg of product. Spot samples of refined cottonseed oil from California, USA, contained < 0.03 mg of endrin and < 0.02 mg of delta-ketoendrin (limits of detection) (FAO/WHO, 1971).

One-hundred-and-ten samples of raw oil and of oil at various stages of processing, i.e., neutralized, hydrogenated, decolourized, deodorized, and shortenings, were collected from seven oil processing factories in Iran in 1974. Endrin was found only in raw and neutralized vegetable oils, at concentrations of 0.004–0.005 mg/litre. Raw imported and native oils contained < 0.01 mg/litre, except for native sunflower oil which contained 0.026 mg/litre (Hashemy-Tonkabony & Soleimani-Amiri, 1976).

Endrin was found in 60 samples of six varieties of the major edible oils and oil seeds used in India, including groundnut, sesame, mustard, coconut, and hydrogenated vegetable oils, collected from a market in Lucknow. Vegetable oil contained 6 µg/litre, mustard oil, 72 µg/litre, and sesame oil, 1690 µg/kg. Of the different types of oil seeds, only mustard seed contained endrin, at 22 µg/kg (Dikshith et al., 1989a).

Endrin was found at a mean concentration of 0.184 (0.097–0.288) mg/kg in samples of cod-liver oil analysed in Germany in 1985 (Ali, 1986). No

Environmental levels and human exposure

residue was found in vegetable oils and fats imported into the United Kingdom (detection limits, 0.02 and 0.001 mg/kg, respectively) (Abbot et al., 1969).

5.1.5.6 Animal feed

Residues of endrin in pressed cottonseed cakes arise primarily from the 1–5% of oil left in the cake after extraction. The residues in cakes from Brazil, India, the USA, and Venezuela were mainly < 0.01–0.02 mg/kg product, levels up to 0.08 mg/kg were found occasionally (FAO/WHO, 1971). The mean concentration of endrin in 32 samples of cattle feed from a local market in India was 0.020 mg/kg (range, 0.013–0.027 mg/kg) (Dikshith et al., 1989b). No endrin was found in 79 samples of cattle feed in Pakistan (Parveen & Masud, 1987). Endrin was not present in samples of domestic and imported animal feed analysed in the USA in 1981–86 (Luke et al., 1988).

None of 42 samples of chicken feed collected from 61 farms in 11 districts of Kenya in 1984 contained endrin (Mugambi et al., 1989).

5.1.6 Miscellaneous products

Endrin was found in 5 of 25 tobacco samples imported into Germany at concentrations of 25–50 µg/kg (Cetinkaya, 1988). No endrin was found in cigarettes of 14 brands collected in Finland in 1960–84 (Mussalo-Rauhamaa et al., 1986). An average content of 0.006 µg/cigarette (range, none detected to 0.02 µg/cigarette) was found in Switzerland (Zimmerli & Marek, 1973).

When raw cotton imported into Germany from 15 countries was analysed, endrin was found in samples from the USSR and Mexico at a concentration of 3 µg/kg (Cetinkaya & Schenek, 1987).

5.2 Exposure of the general population

5.2.1 Total-diet studies

Studies on complete prepared meals in the USA, started in May 1961 and continued to the present, have shown the occasional presence of small amounts of endrin (Williams, 1964; Cummings, 1965, 1966; Duggan et al., 1966, 1967; Martin & Duggan, 1968; Corneliussen, 1969, 1970, 1972;

Manske & Corneliussen, 1974; Manske & Johnson, 1975; Johnson & Manske, 1976, 1977; Manske & Johnson, 1977; Johnson et al., 1981a, 1984). These measurements indicate that the total average daily intake of endrin from food decreased from 0.009 µg/kg body weight in 1965 to 0.0005 µg/kg body weight in 1970 (Duggan & Lipscomb, 1969; Duggan & Corneliussen, 1972), with a further decrease subsequently. In total-diet studies of adults in the USA, representative foods were purchased in 27 US cities in 1980–82; the daily intake of endrin was found to be < 0.001 µg/kg body weight in 1978, but none was detected in 1979, 1980, or 1981–82 (Gartrell et al., 1986a).

Further studies involved retail purchase of 234 food items representative of the total diet of eight US population groups in 1982–84 and preparing them for consumption. The daily intake of endrin in the groups, which included people aged 6–11 months, 2 years, 14–16 years (females), 14–16 years (males), 25–30 years (females), 25–30 years (males), 60–65 years (females), and 60–65 years (males), was 0.1–0.2 ng/kg body weight (FDA, 1988; Gunderson, 1988).

Endrin was not present in the total diets of infants and toddlers in the USA during 1974–75 (Johnson et al., 1979). It was found in one infant food sample at 0.011 mg/kg and in one sample of toddler food at 0.009 mg/kg of food in a study in 1975–76 (Johnson et al., 1981b). Very low residue levels were found occasionally in market-basket samples representing the average 2-week diets of infants (98 samples) and toddlers (110 samples) collected in 10 cities in four geographic areas of the USA in 1977–78 (Podrebarac, 1984). In total-diet studies of infants and toddlers in the USA, representative foods were purchased in 13 US cities in 1980-82; the daily intake of endrin by infants was found to be < 0.001 µg/kg body weight in 1978, and that by toddlers, < 0.001 µg/kg body weight in 1979, but none was detected in the other years (Gartrell et al., 1986b).

Fresh food was bought from four retail grocery stores in Toronto, Canada, in 1985 and combined in five food composites: fresh meat and eggs, root vegetables (including potatoes), fresh fruit, leafy and other surface vegetables, and cows' milk. The concentrations of endrin in the five composites were used to estimate the annual dietary intake of endrin from products in Ontario. Endrin was detected in all composites except eggs and meat; the concentrations were 0.32 µg/kg in leafy vegetables, 0.27 µg/kg in fruit, 0.37 µg/kg in root vegetables, and 0.27 µg/kg in milk. The total annual intake was estimated to be 31.8 µg/person (Davies, 1988).

Environmental levels and human exposure

In a total-diet study carried out in the United Kingdom in 1985–88, 25 samples were obtained in 1984–85 which comprised the 16 food groups considered most likely to contain residues of organochlorine compounds. No endrin was detected (limit of detection, 0.001–0.02 mg/kg, depending on the food group). Endrin was also not detected (< 0.01 mg/kg) in 176 samples of pulses purchased from retail outlets in 1986–87, except in 3 of 20 samples of mung beans in which a mean value of < 0.01 mg/kg (range, none detected to 0.06 mg/kg) was found (United Kingdom Ministry of Agriculture, Fisheries and Food, 1989). No endrin was detected in complete prepared meals during surveys in the United Kingdom in 1965 (Robinson & McGill, 1966; McGill & Robinson, 1968). Similar results were obtained in Switzerland in 1973 (Zimmerli & Marek, 1973), and very low levels were found in two of 73 samples analysed in 1985 (Wüthrich et al., 1985). No endrin residues were found in total-diet studies carried out in the Netherlands in 1976–78 (De Vos et al., 1984).

5.2.2 Levels in human tissues

Although the concentrations of many chlorinated hydrocarbon insecticides, such as DDT, dieldrin, hexachlorocyclohexanes, and hexachlorobenzene, and of their metabolites in blood or adipose tissue of the general population or of occupationally exposed workers have been found to be an excellent index of the level of exposure of the general population, this is not the case for endrin, because it is eliminated rapidly.

5.2.2.1 Adipose tissue

Except in a few cases, endrin was not demonstrated in adipose tissue samples from the general population in the USA in 1962–66 (Hoffman et al., 1964, 1967), 1964 (Hayes et al., 1965; Zavon et al., 1965), 1970–74 (Kutz et al., 1979a,b), and 1975–79 (US EPA, 1983); Canada in 1967–68 (Kadis et al., 1970); Mexico in 1975 (Albert et al., 1980); Argentina in 1968–69; (Wassermann et al., 1969); Belgium in 1968–69 (Wit, 1971); the United Kingdom in 1961 (Hunter et al., 1963), 1964 (Robinson et al., 1965), and 1965–67 (Egan et al., 1965; Abbott et al., 1968, 1972); the Netherlands in 1969 (Wit, 1971); Switzerland in 1972 (Zimmerli & Marek, 1973); Germany in 1970 (Acker & Schulte, 1974); France in 1971 (Fournier et al., 1972); Spain in 1978 (Herrera Marteache et al., 1978); India in 1964 (Dale et al., 1965); or Western Australia in 1965–66 (Wassermann et al., 1968).

No endrin was found in 91 samples of adipose tissue obtained at autopsy in Kingston, Ontario, Canada, in 1979 and 1981 or in 84 samples from Ottawa in 1980 and 1981 (Williams et al., 1984), or in adipose tissue obtained at autopsy from 92 males and 49 females in Ontario municipalities in 1984 (limit of detection, 2.4 µg/kg) (Williams et al., 1988).

These results indicate that endrin is either absent or present at very low levels in the adipose tissue of the general population. It is therefore surprising that Kanitz & Castello (1966) reported the presence of endrin in nine adipose tissue samples from Liguria, Italy, at a mean concentration of 0.93 mg/kg of tissue. The highest concentration was 2.49 mg/kg. Pavan et al. (1987) found endrin at 0.1 and 0.3 mg/kg in 2 of 92 samples of adipose tissue obtained at surgery from people living in the Province of Turin, Italy. In areas where endrin has been used extensively, however, such as India and the lower Mississippi, it has never been found in human adipose tissue (Brooks, 1974).

One of 62 adipose tissue samples obtained at surgery from people in Ciudad Juarez, Mexico, in 1977–78 contained endrin at 0.02 mg/kg (Redetzke et al., 1983).

5.2.2.2 Organs

In samples of liver, kidney, gonad, and brain obtained from the general population of Alberta (Canada), no residue of endrin was detected (Kadis et al., 1970).

5.2.2.3 Blood

No endrin was detected (limit of detection, 0.01 mg/kg) in 4000 blood samples from the general US population in 1976–80 (US E P A, 1983), or in areas where endrin has been used extensively, such as India and the lower Mississippi (Brooks, 1974), or in 26 blood samples from the general population in Nigeria (Atuma, 1985).

5.2.2.4 Breast milk

Endrin was not detected in breast milk in studies in the USA in 1966–78 (Strassman & Kutz, 1977; Currie et al., 1979; Kutz et al., 1979a; Barnett et al., 1979), in El Salvador and Guatemala (De Campos & Olszyna-Marzys, 1979), in Belgium, Italy, and The Netherlands (Kanitz & Castello,

Environmental levels and human exposure

1966; Hendrickx & Maes, 1969; Wegman & Greve, 1974), and in Japan (Yakushiji et al., 1979). No endrin was detected (< 0.01 mg/litre) in 50 breast milk samples from mothers (aged 18–32 years) in Leiden, The Netherlands, in 1969 (Tuinstra, 1971). It was found in one of 12 samples from mothers aged 21–37 in Pavia, Italy, in 1988, at a concentration of 0.01 µg/kg of whole milk, but not in four samples collected in Crotone, southern Italy (Bianchi et al., 1988).

5.2.2.5 Appraisal of exposure of the general population

The occasional presence of low concentrations of endrin in the air of areas where endrin is used in agriculture cannot be considered a significant source of contamination for the general public. The very low concentrations that have been found in surface and drinking-water are also of little significance for public health.

The source of exposure that may be relevant is dietary intake. Apart from accidental contamination, however, intake of endrin by the general population in the countries examined has been and is still far below the maximum acceptable daily intake of 0.2 µg/kg body weight established by the Joint FAO/WHO Meeting in 1970 (FAO/WHO, 1971). This applies equally to the total intake, when the intake from dietary sources is added to that from air and water.

Endrin has not been demonstrated in the large number of samples of organs, adipose tissue, blood, and breast milk analysed in different countries, even in areas where endrin is or was used extensively.

5.3 Occupational exposure during manufacture, formulation and use

5.3.1 Manufacture and formulation

Endrin has not been detected in the blood, plasma, or urine of workers exposed occupationally to endrin (Hayes & Curley, 1968; Jager, 1970). Endrin was detected in blood only after accidental over-exposure. Jager (1970) estimated that the threshold level of endrin in the blood, below which signs or symptoms of intoxication do not occur, lies between 0.05 and 0.10 mg/litre. He estimated the half-life of endrin in the blood to be in the order of 24 h.

The total exposure of workers in a manufacturing and formulation plant was estimated on the basis of determinations of the quantity of the endrin metabolite *anti*-12-hydroxyendrin in urine. Urine of workers exposed to endrin for seven days had concentrations of up to 360 μg/g of creatinine; no unchanged endrin was found. Assuming an average daily excretion of 1.5 g creatinine per day, the total daily excretion of *anti*-12-hydroxyendrin in the urine may be up to 540 μg. This gives a minimal absorption of 0.5 mg endrin, indicating that inhalation of dusts and absorption through the skin may be significant during occupational exposures in manufacture. It is not unreasonable to assume that, as in other species, approximately half of all the endrin absorbed is excreted in the urine as *anti*-12-hydroxyendrin, since both endrin and this metabolite are present in the faeces of workers (Ottevanger & Van Sittert, 1979; Baldwin & Hutson, 1980). Thus, 1 mg/day may be the more accurate figure for exposure in this manufacturing plant. The concentration of *anti*-12-hydroxyendrin in urine decreased more slowly than the concentrations of endrin in blood, with a half-life of 55–75 h (Van Sittert, 1985).

5.3.2 Application

Endrin is applied in agriculture by high-pressure spraying with a hand gun, spraying orchards with a power air blast or boom to control mice, dusting potatoes, spraying row crops, or application from aircraft. These methods of application result in dermal and respiratory exposures.

The potential dermal and respiratory exposure of workers applying endrin formulations in the field has been quantified in a few studies. Respiratory exposure to endrin during spraying of orchards, high-pressure spraying of crops, and piloting of aircraft varied from 0.01 to 0.14 mg/h; dermal exposure during such activities was 0.01–1.64 mg/h. The activity that caused the most exposure was dusting potatoes, which was associated with a respiratory exposure of 0.41 mg/h and a dermal exposure of 18.7 mg/h. Total exposure, calculated as a percentage of a toxic dose/h = {dermal exposure (mg/h) + [respiratory exposure (mg/h) × 10]} ÷ [dermal LD_{50} (mg/kg) × 70] × 100, was 0.21–1.5% (Durham & Wolfe, 1962) (see Table 11). These figures show that although endrin is acutely highly toxic it can be used safely when reasonable precautions are taken (Wolfe et al., 1963; Jegier, 1964; Wolfe et al., 1967; Hayes, 1975).

Endrin was not found in the blood of 20 pesticide sprayers or in 19 controls in Choluteca, southern Honduras (Steinberg et al., 1989).

Environmental levels and human exposure

Table 11. Studies on potential exposure of agricultural workers to endrin, using direct methods

Activity	Exposure		Dermal (mg/h)	Total[a] (%) toxic dose/h	Reference
	Respiratory				
	mg/m³	mg/h			
Spraying orchard cover crops for mouse control		0.01[b]	2.6	0.21	Wolfe et al. (1963)
High-pressure hand-gun spraying orchard cover crops for mouse control		0.01[b]	3	0.25	Wolfe et al. (1967)
Operating air-blast or boom sprayers treating orchard cover crops for mouse control		0.01[b]	2.5	0.21	Wolfe et al. (1967)
Dusting potatoes		0.41[b]	18.7	1.5	Wolfe et al. (1963)
Spraying row crops		ND[b,c]	0.15	(0.01)[d]	Jegier (1964)
Piloting during air application of spray	0.05	0.08[b]	1.18	0.29 (0.16)[e]	Jegier (1964)

[a]For a 70-kg man on the basis of dermal LD_{50} for male rats (18 mg/kg body weight) using the formula given by Durham & Wolfe (1962)
[b]Measured by respirator pad
[c]Not detected
[d]Original values calculated on the basis of maximal exposure; recalculated values shown in parentheses are based on mean exposure.
[e]Calculation based on published data on dermal and respiratory exposure (note in Wolfe et al., 1967)

5.3.3 Appraisal of occupational exposure

No residues were found in healthy workers. The range of threshold levels of endrin in blood below which no sign or symptom of intoxication occurs has been estimated to be 50–100 µg/litre. The half-life of endrin in blood may be in the order of 24 h following occupational exposure. The concentration of *anti*-12-hydroxyendrin in the urine decreased more slowly than the concentration of endrin in blood, with a half-life of 55–75 h.

6. KINETICS AND METABOLISM

6.1 Absorption, distribution, and elimination

6.1.1 *Laboratory animals*

6.1.1.1 *Oral administration*

Rat: One male rat was fed ^{14}C-endrin at a level of 30 mg/kg of diet for 8 days. About 60–70% was excreted on the first day; after three days, the faeces contained more then 80% of the administered radiolabel; by day 9, 84% had been excreted; and there appeared to be a level of saturation after 6–7 days of feeding. Only 0.5% was found in the urine. About 75–80% of the label in the faeces was in at least two different metabolites. The adipose tissue stored 3–4 mg/kg, giving a storage rate of about 10 (FAO/WHO, 1971).

After female rats were given a single oral dose of ^{14}C-endrin at 16, 64, or 128 µg/kg body weight, excretion was rapid. The biological half-life of the doses of 16 and 64 µg/kg was 1–2 days; however, that of 128 µg/kg was approximately 6 days, showing that excretion of higher doses is slower (Korte et al., 1970).

Six CFE rats of each sex were treated with a single oral dose of 0.5 mg ^{14}C-endrin in arachis oil (approximately equivalent to 2.5–3.0 mg/kg body weight), and the radiolabel excreted in urine and faeces was measured over 3 days. The animals were then killed and the radiolabel measured in tissues. A sex difference was noted in the rate of elimination in faeces: 66% of the dose was excreted in 3 days by males and 37% by females; excretion was slower in females but tended to increase daily between days 1 and 3. Small quantities of radiolabel were excreted in the urine, females excreting three times more than males. No radiolabel was found in exhaled air (Hutson et al., 1975). The results are summarized in Tables 12 and 13.

Three rats of each sex were each given a single oral dose of 8 µg ^{14}C-endrin in peanut oil (by gavage) daily for 12 days. A steady state (at which the excreted amount equalled the daily intake) was reached after about 6 days. Females stored about twice as much (27%) as males (14%). The radiolabel was excreted mainly in the faeces: after the first 24 h, 70–75% of the radiolabel was found in faeces as hydrophilic metabolites;

subsequently, only metabolites were present. Four days after the last dose, males retained only 5% and females 15% of the administered radiolabel (Klein et al., 1968; Korte et al., 1970).

Table 12. Rates of excretion of radiolabel by rats treated with a single oral dose of ^{14}C-endrin (percentage of radioactivity administered)

Sex	Urine			Faeces		
	Day 1	Day 2	Day 3	Day 1	Day 2	Day 3
Male	1.3	0.6	0.6	30.6	14.4	21.2
Female	1.8	2.5	2.9	2.3	10.7	24.2

Table 13. Recovery of radiolabel in rat tissues 3 days after a single oral dose of ^{14}C-endrin (percentage of radioactivity administered)

Sex	Urine	Faeces	Liver	Kidneys	Fat	Skin	Remaining carcass	Total
Males	2.7	66.2	1.2	0.6	1.7	2.3	12.2	86.9
Females	7.5	37.2	2.0	0.4	8.0	4.0	28.1	87.2

Rabbit: A Dutch strain male rabbit was given two oral doses of 4.7 mg ^{14}C-endrin in olive oil at an interval of 14 days. Between days 1 and 13, 37% of the first dose was excreted in the urine and 49% in the faeces; the second dose was eliminated similarly. By day 49, 50% had been excreted in urine and 47% in faeces. Faecal excretion was rapid, being almost complete within 24 h, and consisted virtually entirely of unchanged endrin. The urine contained only metabolites (Bedford et al., 1975a). The excretion of metabolites in rabbits thus appears to differ considerably from that in rats: approximately half of a dose of ^{14}C-endrin is excreted in the urine of rabbits and approximately 2% in rats; endrin metabolites are excreted in rat faeces over several days (after a single oral dose), whereas in rabbits faecal excretion is rapid, being almost complete within 24 h, and consists virtually entirely of unchanged endrin. The probable explanation is that the molecular weight threshold for biliary secretion of anions is 325 ± 50 in rats and 475 ± 50 in rabbits (Hirom et al., 1972). The glucuronide and sulfate conjugates of monohydroxyendrin have molecular weights of 572 and 470, respectively. Therefore, conjugates of the endrin metabolites are eliminated in the bile and faeces of rats and in the urine in rabbits.

Kinetics and metabolism

Dog: Three beagles were fed a diet containing endrin at a concentration equivalent to 0.1 mg/kg body weight for 128 days; two other animals were used as controls. The concentration of endrin in blood was determined at weekly intervals. The time to reach a plateau in blood was less than 1 week, and no significant increase in the concentration of endrin in blood was found during this period. The average concentration between day 9 and day 128 was 4 µg/litre. The concentration of endrin in eight organs and tissues of dogs killed 7 days after termination of exposure was < 0.2 mg/kg of tissue; except that the spleen of one dog contained 2.6 mg/kg, and adipose tissue contained 0.2-0.8 mg/kg (Richardson et al., 1967).

6.1.1.2 Intravenous administration

Mouse: The concentrations of endrin were determined in tissues from groups of five adult male CFI mice given endrin intravenously at 5 mg/kg body weight (LD_{90}) in dimethyl sulfoxide. The concentrations prior to convulsions (about 10 min after injection) were approximately 60 mg/kg in liver, 20 mg/kg in brain and omental fat, and approximately 5 mg/litre in blood. The concentration in whole brain 15 min after an intravenous dose of 1.5 mg/kg body weight (the dose that caused ataxia in 90% of animals; TD_{90}) was 9.4 mg/kg. No endrin was detected in the bile of animals with a bile fistula dosed intravenously with the TD_{90} in samples collected after 0.5, 1, or 2 h (Walsh & Fink, 1972).

Rat: Male Holtzman rats with or without a bile fistula were given a single intravenous dose of ^{14}C-endrin at 0.25 m/kg body weight. More than 90% of the excreted radiolabel was found in the faeces of intact animals over the 7-day period after dosing or in the bile of animals with fistulas over 4 days. The mean total percentage recovery of administered radiolabel in faeces, urine, and carcasses was 97% from intact animals 7 days after dosing, and 94% from animals with a bile fistula 4 days after dosing (Cole et al., 1970). No unchanged endrin was found in bile; the major metabolite was *anti*-12-hydroxyendrin (see section 6.2.1).

Rapid excretion was observed in rats given two intravenous injections of ^{14}C-endrin at 0.1 mg/kg body weight at an interval of 4 days. Excretion of the radiolabel was exponential and occurred mainly with faeces; only hydrophilic metabolites were present. With a dose of 200 µg/kg body weight, male rats retained 5.2% and females 12.1% of the administered dose 20 days after the second injection. The biological half-life of endrin after a single intravenous dose of 200 µg/kg body weight was 2.5–3 days in male rats and 4 days in females (Klein et al., 1968; Korte et al., 1970; Brooks, 1974).

Rabbit: When rabbits were given ^{14}C-endrin intravenously, the radiolabel was excreted mainly in the urine and only as metabolites. A probable explanation for the difference in excretion pattern after oral and intravenous administration is that much lower doses (micrograms compared with milligrams) were given intravenously (Korte et al., 1970).

6.1.2 Domestic animals

Twelve cows were fed hay from endrin-sprayed alfalfa containing an average of 1.9, 2.8, or 3.7 mg/kg endrin; the average daily intake of individual animals ranged from 0.04 to 0.11 mg/kg body weight. The average concentrations of endrin in the milk were < 0.05, 0.14, and 0.15 mg/litre, respectively. When endrin dissolved in soya bean oil was fed to 11 dairy cows, levels > 1 mg/kg body weight were required in order for significant quantities of endrin to be detected in milk (Ely et al., 1957).

Dairy cows (eight Jerseys and six Guernseys) were fed diets containing endrin at 0, 0.1, 0.25, 0.75, or 2.0 mg/kg of diet for 12 weeks. No residues were found (limit of detection, 0.01 mg/litre) in the milk of animals that received 0.1 mg/kg, but up to 0.02 mg/litre was found in milk of animals fed 0.25 mg/kg and up to 0.04 mg/litre with 0.75 mg/kg of diet; the highest dose resulted in residues in milk of 0.1 mg/litre. The endrin content of brain, heart, liver, kidneys, body fat, and muscles was < 0.1 mg/kg, but renal fat contained up to 0.8 mg/kg (Kiigemagi et al., 1958).

The concentrations of endrin in milk of cows given feed containing endrin at approximately 0.05, 0.14, and 0.30 mg/kg of whole feed for 5 weeks were 0.004, 0.01, and 0.018 mg/litre, respectively (Williams et al., 1964). A steady (plateau) level in milk was reached after about 15 days.

The concentration of endrin in the milk of dairy cows given feed contaminated with relatively low levels of endrin rose rapidly within a few hours to days and levelled off at a plateau characteristic for each concentration in the feed. The average milk:diet ratio for endrin was 0.07 for feed levels of 0.05–0.3 mg/kg of diet (Biehl & Buck, 1987).

Two lactating cows were fed ^{14}C-endrin for 21 days at an overall dietary concentration of 0.1 mg/kg of diet, which was considered to be comparable to the highest dose that cows are likely to receive in cottonseed cake. Excretion of radiolabel in milk, urine, and faeces reached a plateau 4–9 days after start of treatment. Approximately 3% of the radiolabel was excreted in milk, 65% in urine, and 20% in faeces. Unchanged endrin was not found in urine, but about 30% of the radiolabel in faeces and all of the 0.003–0.006 mg/litre found in milk was endrin. The concentration of endrin equivalent residues was 0.001–0.002 mg/kg in meat and 0.02–0.10 mg/kg in fat; most of the radiolabel in fat consisted of endrin (Baldwin et al., 1976).

Steers, hogs, and lambs fed diets containing endrin at 0, 0.1, 0.25, or 0.75 mg/kg of diet for 12 weeks had residues of < 0.1 mg/kg in red meat, liver, and kidneys and of 0.02–0.2 mg/kg in body fat. Feeding endrin at 2 mg/kg of diet to steers for 12 weeks resulted in residues of 0.9 mg/kg in fat and 0.2–0.3 mg/kg in red meat, liver and kidneys (Terriere et al., 1958). The biotransfer factors for endrin in beef and milk were directly proportional to the octanol–water partition coefficients, while the bioconcentration factor for endrin in vegetation was inversely proportional to the square root of the octanol–water partition coefficient (Travis & Arms, 1988).

Six weeks after the start of feeding seven Delaware X New Hampshire male chicks and eight weeks after the start of feeding seven White Leghorn pullets a diet containing endrin at 0.1 mg/kg, the residues in eggs and meat were < 0.1 mg/kg and that in fat, 0.6 mg/kg. At a dietary level of 0.25 mg/kg, the residue levels were 0.2–0.3 mg/kg in eggs, 0.1 mg/kg in breast meat, and about 1 mg/kg in fat. With 0.75 mg/kg of diet, the levels were 0.4 mg/kg in eggs, 0.24 mg/kg in breast meat, and 3.1 mg/kg in fat (Terriere et al., 1959).

^{14}C-Endrin was administered daily in corn oil in gelatin capsules to six laying hens at a concentration equivalent to 0.13 mg/kg of total diet for 21 weeks. Ingestion and elimination in eggs and excreta were almost balanced after about 16 weeks. The residue levels in eggs were 0.11–0.18 mg/kg and were found in the yolk; none of the known metabolites was detected. The levels of endrin equivalent were about 0.01 mg/kg in breast meat and 0.1 mg/kg in leg meat; higher levels were found in the liver (0.47 mg/kg), kidneys (0.17 mg/kg), and fat (1 mg/kg). The residues were accounted for by unchanged endrin, except in the liver and kidneys, where part probably consisted of polar metabolites. About 50% of the administered radiolabel was excreted in the faeces, 10% of which was in unchanged endrin (Baldwin et al., 1976).

6.1.3 Human beings

The concentrations of endrin in the blood of workmen exposed to endrin were generally below the level of detection: endrin was not found in plasma (< 3 µg/litre) or fat (< 0.03 mg/kg) of workers exposed to endrin for an average of 88 days (Hayes & Curley, 1968). No endrin was found in the blood of healthy people working in an endrin manufacturing plant between 1964 and 1970, at an initial limit of detection of 10 µg/litre, improved after 1965 to 5 µg/litre (Jager, 1970).

Residues of endrin have been found in blood only in individuals with signs of recent intoxication or who have recently had excessive exposure (see section 9.2.2). Endrin appears to be eliminated rapidly from the human body.

6.1.4 Systems in vitro

Isolated liver preparations from Holtzman rats were perfused with a solution containing ^{14}C-endrin at 0.003 mg/ml. Within 1 h, 50% of the radiolabel appeared in the bile; and in 6 h, more than 90% of the total label was found (Cole et al., 1970). With the same dose, radiolabel appeared 2–12 times faster in the bile of livers isolated from male rats as in that of livers from females, which may account for the lower toxicity and lower storage of endrin in adipose tissue in male rats (Klevay, 1971). After perfusion of albino rat liver with a physiological solution containing 40 µg of ^{14}C-endrin, both endrin and hydrophilic metabolites were found (Altmeier & Korte, 1969).

6.2 Biotransformation

Information on the metabolism of endrin up to 1967 was reviewed (Soto & Deichmann, 1967; Brooks, 1969).

6.2.1 Experimental animals

A number of investigations have been carried out since 1970 to elucidate the identity of several metabolites of endrin in rats (Baldwin et al., 1970; Richardson et al., 1970; Hutson et al., 1975; Bedford & Hutson, 1976), rabbits (Bedford et al., 1975a; Hutson, 1981), cows and chickens (Baldwin et al., 1976). The 12-hydroxy derivative was reported to be

Kinetics and metabolism

present in the faeces of rats (Baldwin et al., 1970), and the hydroxyl group was assigned tentatively as *syn* to the epoxide ring. The stereochemical configuration was subsequently shown to be *anti* to the epoxide group (Baldwin et al., 1973), and this configuration was confirmed by the synthesis of *anti*-12-hydroxyendrin (also called 9-*anti*-hydroxyendrin) (Bedford & Harrod, 1973; Bedford et al., 1986a). The chemical structures of these compounds are shown in Figure 2; the chemical names are given in Annex I.

Formation of *anti*-12-hydroxyendrin (*III*), together with its sulfate and glucuronide conjugates, is considered to be the major route of metabolism of endrin. Four other metabolites have been reported, but their concentrations are generally smaller than that of *anti*-12-hydroxyendrin and its conjugates. These four metabolites are *syn*-12-hydroxyendrin (*II*; tentative identification), 3-hydroxyendrin (*IV*; synthesized and structure confirmed by Bedford et al., 1986b), 12-ketoendrin (*V*), and the product of formal hydroxylation of endrin, the 4,5-*trans*-dihydroisodrindiol (*VI*; tentative structure). The *trans*-diol (*VI*) is a minor metabolite in both rats and rabbits; it may be formed via an oxidation–reduction pathway involving intermediates of the corresponding ketol (*VII*). Each of the hydroxy compounds is also excreted partly as its sulfate or glucuronide in the urine of animals (Bedford et al., 1975a,b; Hutson et al., 1975).

The three monohydroxylated derivatives of endrin, *syn*- and *anti*-12-hydroxyendrin (*II* and *III*) and 3-hydroxyendrin (*IV*), are the products of the action of liver microsomal monooxygenases on endrin (Bedford & Hutson, 1976). These alcohols are also conjugated to glucuronides and sulfates to some extent in the liver. Comparative metabolic studies with rat liver microsome preparations have shown that free *syn*-12-hydroxyendrin, but not its free *anti*-isomer, is the precursor of 12-ketoendrin (*V*) (Hutson & Hoadley, 1974).

Rats exhibit a sex difference in the rate of metabolism. The major metabolite in animals of each sex is *anti*-12-hydroxyendrin, which is excreted via the bile as the glucuronide; this undergoes enterohepatic circulation and is eliminated as the aglycone in the faeces, together with two minor metabolites, 3-hydroxyendrin and 4,5-*trans*-dihydroisodrindiol. Male rats produce the metabolite at a higher rate than do females. The major urinary metabolite in male CFE rats was 12-ketoendrin, while females excreted mainly *anti*-12-hydroxyendrin *O*-sulfate. Endrin and the lipophilic metabolite 12-ketoendrin were the major compounds found in the organs and tissues of male and female CFE rats 3 days after a single oral

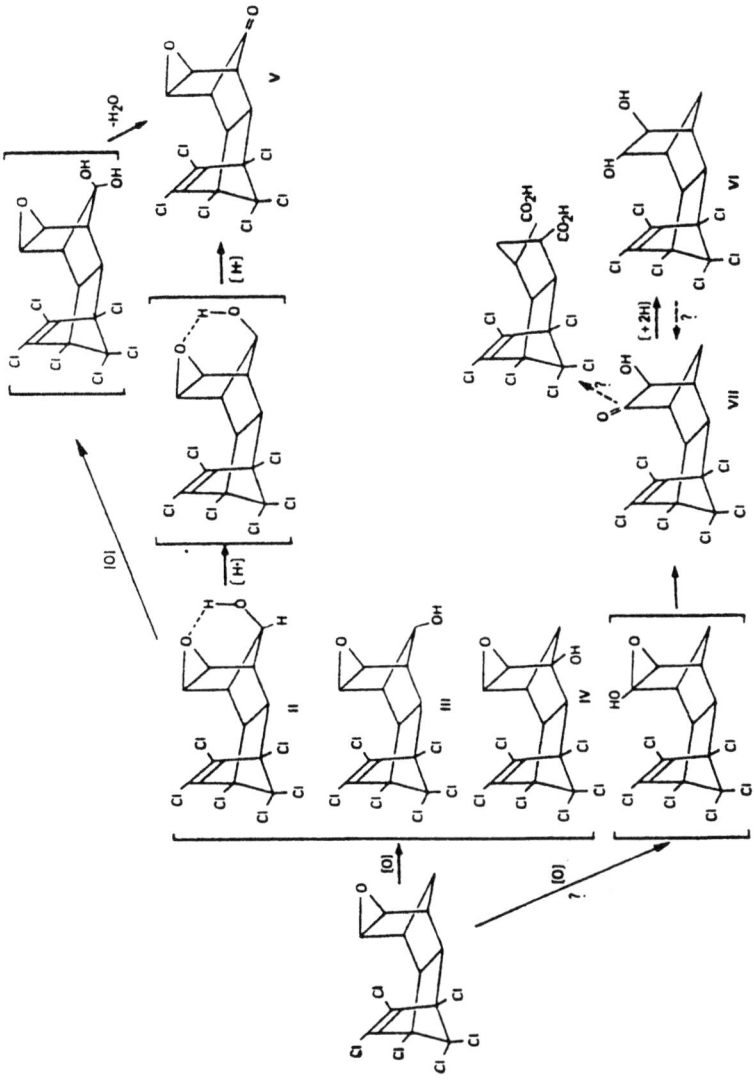

Fig. 2. Mechanisms of biotransformation of endrin (*I*) (see also Annex I)

Kinetics and metabolism

dose of endrin, but the ratio of endrin:12-ketoendrin was 2/1 in females and 1/8 in males. Thus, 12-ketoendrin constituted most of the radiolabel in the liver and kidneys of males and endrin that in the kidneys of females (Hutson et al., 1975; Hutson, 1981).

The metabolism of endrin in rabbits is superficially different from that in rats. The major metabolite is still *anti*-12-hydroxyendrin, but it is conjugated with sulfate and eliminated in the urine. Some *syn*-12-hydroxyendrin was also detected as its sulfate in urine, and perhaps conjugation and elimination prevented further oxidation to 12-ketoendrin. The respective glucuronide conjugates were also eliminated in the urine, as were the glucuronides of 3-hydroxyendrin and the 4,5-*trans*-diol (*VI*) (Bedford et al., 1975b; Hutson, 1981).

Studies with ^{14}C-endrin in lactating cows showed that the residues in milk and body fat consisted of unchanged endrin, although traces of 12-ketoendrin were consistently found in fat. As in rats, *anti*-12-hydroxyendrin was the major metabolite in urine and faeces, the urine being the major excretory route, as in rabbits. 12-Ketoendrin and *syn*-12-hydroxyendrin were minor metabolites in cow urine (Baldwin et al., 1976). Thus, although the metabolic pathways of endrin in cows are qualitatively similar to those in rats and rabbits, quantitative differences are seen in faecal and urinary excretion.

In hens, only endrin was found as a residue in meat, fat, and eggs. Unchanged endrin accounted for about 10% of the radiolabel in excreta, and the major metabolite was *anti*-12-hydroxyendrin and its sulfate conjugate. No 12-ketoendrin was detected in tissues, eggs, or excreta. The metabolism of endrin in hens is fundamentally similar to that in rats, rabbits, and cows, except that they produce neither *syn*-12-hydroxyendrin nor the related 12-ketoendrin. The rate of metabolism, however, was much lower than in cows (Baldwin et al., 1976). The absence of 12-ketoendrin in birds was confirmed in a study of four species killed by endrin (Stickel et al., 1979). Hutson et al. (1975) suggested that the acute toxicity of endrin in birds is not associated with the formation of 12-ketoendrin.

6.2.2   Human beings

No endrin was found (limit of detection, 0.0016 mg/litre) in 14 samples of urine from workers exposed to aldrin, dieldrin, and endrin, even though workers with a complete work history had been exposed to endrin for an average of 2160 h (Hayes & Curley, 1968). Endrin was not detected in urine from five men and five women (Cueto & Hayes, 1962; Cueto & Biros, 1967). No unchanged endrin was found in the urine of Dutch workers exposed to endrin, but it occurred in the faeces (Jager, 1970; Baldwin & Hutson, 1980).

Neither 3-hydroxyendrin nor the diol was detected in urine or faeces (Hutson, 1981). *anti*-12-Hydroxyendrin was present in the urine of workers exposed to endrin, and the glucuronide was found in the faeces. Concentrations of up to 0.36 mg/g of creatinine were found in urine after 7 days, accompanied by a sharp rise in the level of D-glutaric acid (excreted in the urine of mammals as a metabolite of D-glucuronolactone [Marsh, 1963]), indicating that liver enzyme induction may have occurred. The levels tended to decrease over the weekend (Ottevanger & Van Sittert, 1979). Endrin, *anti*-12-hydroxyendrin, 12-ketoendrin, and the beta-glucuronide of *anti*-12-hydroxyendrin were not found in the blood of workers at a Dutch plant for the manufacture of endrin (limit of detection, 2 µg/litre). Both endrin and *anti*-12-hydroxyendrin were found in the faeces, and all urine samples contained the beta-glucuronide of *anti*-12-hydroxyendrin up to a concentration of 0.14 mg/litre as *anti*-12-hydroxyendrin (Baldwin & Hutson, 1980).

Hydroxylation at *anti*-C-12 is relatively rapid and accounts for the rapid metabolism of endrin. Even *syn*-12-hydroxyendrin is hydroxylated rapidly at its *anti*-C-12 position, affording 12-ketoendrin (Hutson, 1981).

As neither endrin nor its metabolites were found in the blood of exposed, healthy workers, exposure can be measured by determining *anti*-12-hydroxyendrin in urine. A quantitative relationship between exposure to endrin and the concentration of this metabolite cannot be established, however, owing to lack of data.

6.2.3 *Microorganisms*

In mixed anaerobic microbial populations developed using inocula from soil, freshwater mud, sheep rumen, and chicken litter, endrin (like other cyclodiene compounds) was monodechlorinated at the methylene bridge carbon atom. Neither endrin nor any other compound was further metabolized. The 10 obligate anaerobic bacteria that made up the mixed population were subsequently isolated in pure culture. Of these, only *Clostridium bifermentans*, *C. glycolium*, and other *Clostridium* species

Kinetics and metabolism

were capable of dehalogenation, but at a rate that was much slower than that of the mixed population (Maule et al., 1987).

6.2.4 Plants

Three experiments were carried out on tobacco plants. In the first experiment, 2.08 mg of ^{14}C-endrin were applied to the leaves with free aeration during the experimental period. In the second test, the same dose was applied but with little aeration; and in the third, plants were exposed to 1.04 mg of ^{14}C-endrin with little aeration. An initial residue level of 50–100 mg/kg was found on leaves in all three experiments, but, subsequently, less residue was found on plants with free aeration. Six weeks after treatment, 30–47% of radiolabel was recovered in residues, which consisted of endrin and hydrophilic substances (Weisgerber et al., 1969; Donoso et al., 1979).

The leaves of cotton plants were treated with 4.2 mg of ^{14}C-endrin, and the application was repeated after 2 and again after 6 weeks, at which time parathion was also applied. At harvest, two-thirds of the radiolabel had evaporated, and the total residue in cotton seed was 0.333 mg/kg. Endrin and two groups of degradation products were found in the plants; one of these products (possibly delta-ketoendrin) was only slightly more hydrophilic than endrin, and the other was very hydrophilic. Most of the metabolites were found on the surface of the leaves. When delta-ketoendrin was applied to white cabbage, it disappeared more slowly than endrin, with the formation of hydrophilic metabolites (Korte, 1969).

7. EFFECTS ON ORGANISMS IN THE ENVIRONMENT

7.1 Microorganisms

The interactions of halogenated pesticides and microorganisms have been reviewed extensively (Pfister, 1972).

In three Willamette valley soils (USA) treated with endrin at 0, 1 or 10 mg/kg, no effect was found 30 days after application on the function and activity of the microbial population, the decomposition of native organic matter, the transformation of native soil nitrogen, ammonification of peptone, or nitrification of ammonium sulphate (Bollen & Tu, 1971). Even at an annual application rate of 5 lb/acre (5.6 kg/ha) for 5 years, no effect was seen on the numbers or kinds of soil fungi, the numbers of bacteria, the decomposition rate of organic matter (measured by CO_2 production), or the oxidation of ammonium to nitrate (Martin et al., 1959).

Endrin at a concentration of 100 mg/kg of soil had no effect on denitrification in soil under anaerobic incubation for 5 days at 30 °C or in an isolated denitrifying bacterium (Bollag & Henninger, 1976). A concentration of 1000 mg/kg had no effect on methanogenesis, sulfate reduction, or carbon dioxide evolution in anaerobic salt-marsh sediments (Kiene & Capone, 1984).

The growth rates of two strains of blue-green algae were decreased in the presence of endrin at a concentration of 0.29 µg/litre (Batterton et al., 1971), and the productivity of many forms of natural phytoplankton in estuarine waters was decreased by 46% when they were exposed to 1 mg/litre (Butler, 1963).

7.2 Aquatic organisms

7.2.1 Invertebrates

Acute toxicity of endrin to invertebrates is given in Tables 14 and 15.

A static system was used to study the toxicity of endrin to a polychaete worm (*Nereis virens*) in water and sediment, in which sea water or sediment (containing 17% sand, 83% clay, and 2% organic carbon) was

Effects on organisms in the environment

Table 14. Acute toxicity of endrin to freshwater invertebrates

Organism	Size/age	Static/flow[a]	Temp. (°C)	Hardness (mg CaCO$_3$/l)	pH	Parameter	Concentration (mg/l)	Reference
Red snail *Indoplanorbis exustus*		Static				48-h LC$_{50}$	7200	Hashimoto & Nishiuchi (1981)
Marsh snail *Semisulcospira libertina*		Static				48-h LC$_{50}$	9500	Hashimoto & Nishiuchi (1981)
Snail *Physa acuta*		Static				48-h LC$_{50}$	12 000	Hashimoto & Nishiuchi (1981)
Water flea *Daphnia magna*		Static	18–23			48-h LC$_{50}$	160	Thurston et al.(1985)
		Static	21	44	7.1	48-h LC$_{50}$	4.2	Mayer & Ellersieck (1986)
		Static	18	48	7.4	48-h LC$_{50}$	41–74	Mayer & Ellersieck (1986)
		Static	22–24	240	8.0	96-h LC$_{50}$	59	Elnabarawy et al. (1986)
Water flea *Daphnia pulex*		Static	15	44	7.1	48-h LC$_{50}$	20	Mayer & Ellersieck (1986)
		Static	22–24	240	8.0	96-h LC$_{50}$	30	Elnabarawy et al. (1986)
Water flea *Daphnia reticulata*		Static	22–24	240	8.0	96-h LC$_{50}$	24	Elnabarawy et al. (1986)
Water flea *Simocephalus serrulatus*		Static	21	44	7.1	48-h LC$_{50}$	45	Mayer & Ellersieck (1986)
		Static	15	44	7.1	48-h LC$_{50}$	26	Mayer & Ellersieck (1986)
Water flea *Cypridopsis vidua*	Adult	Static	21	44	7.1	48-h LC$_{50}$	1.8	Mayer & Ellersieck (1986)

Table 14. (contd)

Organism	Size/age	Static/flow[a]	Temp. (°C)	Hardness (mg CaCO$_3$/l)	pH	Parameter	Concentration (mg/l)	Reference
Sow bug (isopod) *Asellus brevicaudus*	Adult	Static	15	44	7.1	96-h LC$_{50}$	1.5	Mayer & Ellersieck (1986)
Scud *Gammarus fasciatus*	Adult Adult	Static Static	21 15	44 272	7.1 7.4	96-h LC$_{50}$ 96-h LC$_{50}$	4.3 1.3	Mayer & Ellersieck (1986) Mayer & Ellersieck (1986)
Scud *Gammarus lacustris*	Adult	Static	21	44	7.1	96-h LC$_{50}$	3.0	Mayer & Ellersieck (1986)
Crayfish *Orconectes nais*	3–5 weeks Adult	Static Static	21 21	272 272	7.4 7.4	96-h LC$_{50}$ 96-h LC$_{50}$	3.2 320	Mayer & Ellersieck (1986) Mayer & Ellersieck (1986)
Crayfish *Orconectes immunis*	0.4–2.0 g	Flow	18–23			96-h LC$_{50}$	> 89	Thurston et al. (1985)
Red crayfish *Procambarus clarki*		Static				48-h LC$_{50}$	300	Muncy & Oliver (1963)
Tantytarsus *Tantytarsus dissimilis*		Static	18–23			48-h LC$_{50}$	0.84	Thurston et al. (1985)
Glass shrimp *Palaemonetes kadiakensis*	Adult Adult	Static Flow	21 21	272 272	7.4 7.4	96-h LC$_{50}$ 96-h LC$_{50}$	3.2 0.5	Mayer & Ellersieck (1986) Mayer & Ellersieck (1986)

Table 14. (contd)

Organism	Size/age	Static/flow[a]	Temp. (°C)	Hardness (mg CaCO$_3$/l)	pH	Parameter	Concentration (mg/l)	Reference
Stonefly *Acroneuria* sp.	Larvae	Static	15	44	7.1	96-h LC$_{50}$	> 0.18	Mayer & Ellersieck (1986)
Stonefly *Claasenia sabulosa*	Larvae	Static	15	44	7.1	96-h LC$_{50}$	0.076	Mayer & Ellersieck (1986)
Stonefly *Pteronarcella badia*	Larvae	Static	15	44	7.1	96-h LC$_{50}$	0.54	Mayer & Ellersieck (1986)
Stonefly *Pteronarcys californica*	Larvae	Static	15	44	7.1	96-h LC$_{50}$	0.25	Mayer & Ellersieck (1986)
Mayfly *Baetis* sp.	Larvae	Static	15	44	7.1	96-h LC$_{50}$	0.9	Mayer & Ellersieck (1986)
Mayfly *Hexagenia bilineata*	Larvae	Static	15	44	7.1	96-h LC$_{50}$	62	Mayer & Ellersieck (1986)
Damselfly *Ischnura verticalis*	Larvae Larvae	Static Static	21 21	44 272	7.1 7.4	96-h LC$_{50}$ 96-h LC$_{50}$	2.4 2.1	Mayer & Ellersieck (1986)
Snipe fly *Atherix variegata*	Larvae	Static	15	44	7.1	96-h LC$_{50}$	4.6	Mayer & Ellersieck (1986)

[a] Static, static conditions (water unchanged for duration of test); flow, flow-through conditions; endrin concentration in water maintained continuously

Table 15. Acute toxicity of endrin to estuarine and marine invertebrates

Organism	Size/age	Static/flow[a]	Temp. (°C)	Salinity (%)	Parameter	Concentration (µg/l)	Reference
Sand shrimp *Crangon septemspinosa*		Static			96-h LC_{50}	1.7	Eisler (1970a)
		Static			96-h LC_{50}	0.2–2.0	McLeese & Metcalfe (1980)
		Static			96-h LC_{50}	4–120	McLeese & Metcalfe (1980)
Brown shrimp *Penaeus aztecus*	Juvenile	Flow	15	26	48-h LC_{50}	0.2	Mayer (1987)
Pink shrimp *Penaeus duorarum*	Juvenile	Flow	17	30	48-h LC_{50}	0.2	Mayer (1987)
	Adult	Flow	17	28	96-h LC_{50}	0.037	
Grass shrimp *Palaemonetes pugio*	Larvae	Flow	25	13	96-h LC_{50}	1.2	Mayer (1987)
	Juvenile	Flow	25	23	96-h LC_{50}	0.35	
	Adult	Flow	25	21	96-h LC_{50}	0.69	
Blue crab *Callinectes sapidus*	Juvenile	Flow	11	16	48-h LC_{50}	15	Mayer (1987)
Hermit crab *Pagurus longicarpus*					96-h LC_{50}	1.2	Eisler (1970a)

[a] Static, static conditions (water unchanged for duration of test); flow, flow-through conditions; endrin concentration in water maintained continuously

present at a temperature of 9–10 °C for 12 days. None of the worms in sea water died after exposure to endrin at 0.11 mg/litre for 12 days, but two of five worms exposed to 28 mg/kg in sediment died in this period (McLeese et al., 1982).

The mean 96-h LC_{50} for the oligochaetes *Stylodrilus heringianus* and *Limnodrilus hoffmeisteri* exposed to sediment from Lake Michigan contaminated with ^{14}C-endrin was 2588 ± 1974 mg/kg dry weight of sediment in four assays and 2725 ± 955 mg/kg in two assays. The toxicity to *L. hoffmeisteri* appeared to be reduced in the presence of *S. heringianus*. The 96-h EC_{50} burrowing avoidance values were 15.3–19 mg/kg for *S. heringianus* and 59 mg/kg of sediment for *L. hoffmeisteri* (Keilty et al., 1988a).

Sediment reworking by *L. hoffmeisteri* alone and with *S. heringianus* was measured by monitoring the burial of a ^{137}Cs marker layer in sediments dosed with ^{12}C- and ^{14}C-endrin at concentrations of 5.5–81 400 µg/kg of dry sediment. With low endrin concentrations, the marker layer burial rate did not suggest stimulation of reworking by either *L. hoffmeisteri* or *S. heringianus*. At higher concentrations, the reworking rates were equal to or slower than control rates at the beginning of the experiment but decreased thereafter. The presence of *S. heringianus* appeared to enhance the reworking response of *L. hoffmeisteri*. A reduction in the post-experimental mortality and an increase in the dry weight of *L. hoffmeisteri* in tests with the two species implies that *L. hoffmeisteri* benefits from the presence of *S. heringianus*, although the reverse was not observed. High concentrations of endrin in the upper 3 cm of the final sediment showed that the worms had transported the contaminant upward. The bioaccumulation factor for *S. heringianus* ranged from 9.7 to 43.8 and was consistently three to four times greater than that for *L. hoffmeisteri* (1.7–13.6) (Keilty et al., 1988b).

The reworking rates of *S. heringianus* in microcosms containing sediments dosed with ^{14}C-endrin at 3.1–42 000 µg/kg of dry matter were measured at 10 °C by monitoring a ^{137}Cs marker layer buried in contaminated and uncontaminated microcosms. Alterations in reworking rates were observed at endrin concentrations 5.5 orders of magnitude below the LC_{50} of 1650 mg/kg. At the lower concentrations, a possible stimulatory effect on the marker layer burial rate in the first 300–600 h was followed by a significant decrease relative to the controls. At the higher concentrations, the rates were equal or slower during the first 600 h and decreased dramatically in the last 600 h. Mortality was 9.3–28% at 11 500 and 42 000 µg/kg and 0–6.7% at all the other concentrations tested, including controls. The dry weights of the worms at the end of the experiment were inversely related to the high concentrations. The bioaccumulation factors ranged from 34 to 67 on the basis of grams of dry organism to grams of dry sediment (Keilty et al., 1988c).

The effect of addition of endrin at 50 mg/kg dry weight of sediment on protein utilization by *S. heringianus* was examined on days 4, 8, 20, 28, 39, and 69. A slight increase in the relative percentage of protein to total body weight was observed, but the authors concluded that estimation of total protein is not a useful measure of sublethal responses (Keilty & Stehly, 1989).

The total organic carbon content of sediment had little apparent effect on the toxicity of endrin in the freshwater amphipod *Hyalella azteca*. The 10-day LC_{50} for endrin in sediment (dry-weight basis) was 4.4 µg/litre at 3.0% total organic carbon and 6.0 µg/litre at 11.2% carbon (Nebeker et al., 1989).

The EC_{50}s in the green sea urchin (*Strongylocentrotus droebachiensis*), the purple sea urchin (*S. purpuratus*), the red sea urchin (*S. franciscanus*), and the sand dollar (*Dendraster excentricus*) were 103–441 µg/litre for sperm in a static system and 221–>362 µg/litre for embryos in a continuous flow of sea water (temperature, 8.2–8.4 °C; salinity, 30.0 parts per thousand; pH 7.8–8.1 for the sea urchins and 12.5–13.0 °C, 30.0 parts per thousand, and pH 8.0–8.1 for sand dollar embryos), both with an exposure time of 120 h. In a larval test of static exposure of Dungeness crab (*Cancer magister*), the EC_{50} was 2.0 µg/litre (Dinnel et al., 1989).

Endrin was tested at 0, 0.025, 0.05, 0.1, 0.25, 0.5, 1.0, 2.5, 5.0, and 10 mg/litre for its effects on embryos of the American oyster (*Crassostrea virginica*) and their larvae. Fertilized eggs were studied after 48 h, and survival and growth of veliger larvae were studied in 2-day old larvae and in larvae kept for a further 12 days at 24 °C. The results varied considerably. The estimated concentration that would cause an approximately 50% reduction in the number of eggs that develop into normal straight-hinge larvae, calculated by interpolation from the data, was 0.79 µg/litre and that at which 50% of the larvae survived was > 10.0 mg/litre (Davis & Hidu, 1969).

Effects on organisms in the environment

In the mysid shrimp *Mysidopsis bahia*, exposed for the complete life cycle, acute lethality (over 96 h) was observed with endrin at 120 ng/litre; increased oxygen consumption was measurable within 24 h of exposure. The lowest-observed-effect level for chronic lethality was 60 ng/litre; sublethal effects on growth (reduced by day 4 of exposure) and oxygen consumption (increased by day 10 of exposure) were observed before death (over 20 days). Reduced reproductive capacity (assessed as production of young) was observed at 30 ng/litre over 20 days—the time to full maturity (McKenney, 1986).

Behavioural changes were observed in stoneflies (*Pteronarcys dorsata*) within 4 days of exposure to 96.1% endrin at 0.07 µg/litre and in caddis flies (*Brachycentrus americanus*) at 0.15 µg/litre. The 28-day LC_{50} was < 0.03 µg/litre for caddis flies and 0.07 µg/litre for stoneflies (Anderson & DeFoe, 1980).

7.2.2 Fish

7.2.2.1 Acute toxicity

Endrin is highly toxic for both freshwater and marine fish. The available data are summarized in Tables 16 and 17.

7.2.2.2 Short-term toxicity

Channel catfish (*Ictalurus punctatus*) were exposed continuously to renewed solutions of endrin in water at 15 and 22 °C. Measured endrin concentrations of 0.25–0.30 µg/litre were found to be acutely toxic to the fish within 10 days or less. None of the fish survived blood concentrations exceeding 0.28 mg/litre, a well-defined threshold concentration of endrin in blood, and none died at less than 0.23 mg/litre. The concentration of endrin in the blood of fish exposed to lethal concentrations in water for periods insufficient to cause death were markedly lower than that in fish that died from exposure to the same water (Mount et al., 1966).

The 28-day LC_{50} for 96.1% eldrin in bullheads (*Ictalurus melas*) was 0.10 µg/litre (Anderson & DeFoe, 1980).

In larval fathead minnows (< 24 h old) exposed continuously to endrin (98%) for 28–30 days in a flow-through system, growth was the most sensitive parameter. A 48-h exposure to 0.62 µg/litre caused significant

Table 16. Acute toxicity of endrin to freshwater fish

Organism	Size/age	Static/flow[a]	Temp. (°C)	Hardness (mg CaCO$_3$/l)	pH	Parameter	Concentration (μ g/l)	Reference
Tilupa sp.		Static	15	44	7.1	96-h LC$_{50}$	12	Mayer & Ellersieck (1986)
Coho salmon *Oncorhynchus kisutch*	1.9 g	Static	16	44	7.1	96-h LC$_{50}$	0.089	Mayer & Ellersieck (1986)
		Static	20			96-h LC$_{50}$	0.27	Katz & Chadwick (1961)
Chinook salmon *Oncorhynchus tshawytscha*	6–8 g	Static	20			96-h LC$_{50}$	0.92	Katz & Chadwick (1961)
Cutthroat trout *Salmo clarki*	1.0 g	Static	13	44	7.1	96-h LC$_{50}$	> 1.0	Mayer & Ellersieck (1986)
Rainbow trout *Oncorhynchus mykiss*	1.0 g	Static	13	44	7.1	96-h LC$_{50}$	0.75	Mayer & Ellersieck (1986)
	1.0 g	Static	13	272	7.4	96-h LC$_{50}$	0.74	
	1.4 g	Static	2	44	7.1	96-h LC$_{50}$	2.4	
	1.4 g	Static	7	44	7.1	96-h LC$_{50}$	1.4	
	1.4 g	Static	13	44	7.1	96-h LC$_{50}$	1.11	
	1.4 g	Static	18	44	7.1	96-h LC$_{50}$	0.75	
	0.6–8.0 g	Flow	18–23			96-h LC$_{50}$	0.3	Thurston et al. (1985)
Goldfish *Carrassius auratus*	1–4 g	Flow	12	314	7.6	96-h LC$_{50}$	0.44	Mayer & Ellersieck (1986)
		Flow	18–23			96-h LC$_{50}$	0.95	Thurston et al. (1985)
		Static				48-h LC$_{50}$	1.0	Hashimoto & Nishiuchi (1981)

Table 16. (contd)

Organism	Size/age	Static/flow[a]	Temp. (°C)	Hardness (mg CaCO$_3$/l)	pH	Parameter	Concentration (μg/l)	Reference
Carp *Cyprinus carpio*		Flow	12	314	7.6	96-h LC$_{50}$	0.32	Mayer & Ellersieck (1986)
		Static				48-h LC$_{50}$	0.84	Hashimoto & Nishiuchi (1981)
Medaka *Oryzias latipes*		Static				48-h LC$_{50}$	1.4	Hashimoto & Nishiuchi (1981)
Pond loach *Misgurnus anguilicaudatus*		Static				48-h LC$_{50}$	4.9	Hashimoto & Nishiuchi (1981)
Fathead minnow *Pimephales promelas*	1.2 g	Static	18	44	7.1	96-h LC$_{50}$	1.8	Mayer & Ellersieck (1986)
	0.9 g	Flow	12	314	7.6	96-h LC$_{50}$	0.24	
		Static				24-h LC$_{50}$	12	Kagan et al. (1986)
	Larvae	Static	25–26	46	7.1–8.3	96-h LC$_{50}$	0.7	Jarvinen et al. (1988)
	0.2–1.0 g	Flow	18–23			96-h LC$_{50}$	0.65	Thurston et al. (1985)
Bluntnose minnow *Pimephales notatus*		Static				96-h LC$_{50}$	0.29	Johnson (1968)
Black bullhead *Ictalurus melas*	1.5 g	Static	24	44	7.1	96-h LC$_{50}$	1.13	Mayer & Ellersieck (1986)
Channel catfish *Ictalurus punctatus*	5.2 g	Static	18	44	7.1	96-h LC$_{50}$	1.9	Mayer & Ellersieck (1986)
	1.4 g	Static	24	44	7.1	96-h LC$_{50}$	0.32	

Table 16. (contd)

Organism	Size/age	Static/flow[a]	Temp. (°C)	Hardness (mg CaCO$_3$/l)	pH	Parameter	Concentration (mg/l)	Reference
Mosquito fish								
Gambusia affinis	0.6 g	Static	17	44	7.1	96-h LC$_{50}$	1.1	Mayer & Ellersieck (1986)
	0.222 g	Static	25			96-h LC$_{50}$	5.27	El-Sebae (1987)
Bluegill								
Lepomis macrochirus	1.5 g	Static	18	44	7.1	96-h LC$_{50}$	0.61	Mayer & Ellersieck (1986)
	0.5 g	Static	18	272	7.4	96-h LC$_{50}$	0.53	
	1.3 g	Static	7	44	7.1	96-h LC$_{50}$	0.73	
	1.3 g	Static	13	44	7.1	96-h LC$_{50}$	0.68	
	1.3 g	Static	18	44	7.1	96-h LC$_{50}$	0.41	
	1.3 g	Static	24	44	7.1	96-h LC$_{50}$	0.37	
	1.3 g	Static	29	44	7.1	96-h LC$_{50}$	0.19	
Largemouth bass								
Micropterus salmoides	2.5 g	Static	18	272	7.4	96-h LC$_{50}$	0.31	Mayer & Ellersieck (1986)
Yellow perch								
Perca flavescens		Flow	12	314	7.6	96-h LC$_{50}$	0.15	Mayer & Ellersieck (1986)
Tilapia								
Tilapia mossambica	1.1 g	Static	24	44	7.1	96-h LC$_{50}$	< 5.6	Mayer & Ellersieck (1986)
Tilapia (Behera strain)	0.825 g	Static	25			96-h LC$_{50}$	10.09	El-Sebae (1987)
Tilapia zilli								

Table 16. (contd)

Organism	Size/age	Static/flow[a]	Temp. (°C)	Hardness (mg CaCO$_3$/l)	pH	Parameter (mg/l)	Concentration (μg/l)	Reference
Tilapia (Alexandria strain) *Tilapia zilli*	0.825 g	Static	25			96-h LC$_{50}$	0.26	El-Sebae (1987)
Guppy *Poecilia reticulata*		Static	20			96-h LC$_{50}$	0.9	Katz & Chadwick (1961)
Flagfish *Jordanella floridae*	2–3 days	Static	24–26	43–48	6.9–7.8	96-h LC$_{50}$	0.85	Hermanutz et al. (1985)

[a] Static, static condition (water unchanged for the duration of the test); flow, flow-through conditions; endrin concentration in water maintained continuously.

Table 17. Acute toxicity of endrin to estuarine and marine fish

Organism	Size/age	Static/flow[a]	Temp. (°C)	Salinity (%)	Parameter	Concentration (µg/l)	Reference
American eel *Anguilla rostrata*	57 mm	Static	20	24	96-h LC_{50}	0.6	Eisler (1970b)
Atlantic riverside *Menidia menidia*	54 mm	Static	20	24	96-h LC_{50}	0.05	Eisler (1970b)
Blue head *Thalassoma bifasciatum*	90 mm	Static	20	24	96-h LC_{50}	0.1	Eisler (1970b)
Gulf menhaden *Brevoortia patronus*	Juvenile	Flow	27	29	24-h LC_{50}	0.8	Mayer (1987)
Sheepshead minnow *Cyprinodon variegatus*	Juvenile	Flow	14	30	48-h LC_{50}	1.0	Mayer (1987)
	Juvenile	Flow	30	24	96-h LC_{50}	0.34	
	Adult	Flow	18	18	96-h LC_{50}	0.38	
	Adult	Flow	30	16	96-h LC_{50}	0.36	
Longnose killifish *Fundulus similis*	Juvenile	Flow	25	19	24-h LC_{50}	0.23	Mayer (1987)
Striped killifish *Fundulus majalis*	40 mm	Static	20	24	96-h LC_{50}	0.3	Eisler (1970b)

Effects on organisms in the environment

Table 17. (contd)

Organism	Size/age	Static/flow[a]	Temp. (°C)	Salinity (%)	Parameter	Concentration (μg/l)	Reference
Mummichog *Fundulus heteroclitus*	51 mm	Static	20	24	96-h LC_{50}	0.6	Eisler (1970b)
Sailfin molly *Poecilia latipinna*	Adult	Flow	20	27	96-h LC_{50}	0.63	Mayer (1987)
Spot *Leiostomus xanthurus*	Juvenile	Flow	12	24	48-h LC_{50}	0.3	Mayer (1987)
Striped mullet *Mugil cephalus*	Juvenile 83 mm	Flow Static	14 20	30 24	48-h LC_{50} 96-h LC_{50}	0.4 0.3	Mayer (1987) Eisler (1970b)
White mullet *Mugil curema*	Juvenile	Flow	29		48-h LC_{50}	2.6	Butler (1963)
Northern puffer *Sphaeroides maculatus*	131 mm	Static	20	24	96-h LC_{50}	3.1	Eisler (1970b)
Striped bass *Morone saxatilis*	2.7 g	Static	16–18	28	96-h LC_{50}	0.09	Korn & Earnest (1974)
Shiner perch *Cymatogaster aggregata*	1.2–11 g 1.2–11 g	Static Int. flow	13 13	26 26	96-h LC_{50} 96-h LC_{50}	0.8 0.12	Earnest & Benville (1972)

Table 17. (contd)

Organism	Size/age	Static/flow[a]	Temp. (°C)	Salinity (%)	Parameter	Concentration(µg/l)	Reference
Dwarf perch *Micrometrus minimus*	1.2–11 g 1.2–11 g	Static Int. flow	13 13	18 28	96-h LC$_{50}$ 96-h LC$_{50}$	0.6 0.13	Earnest & Benville (1972)
Threespine stickleback *Gasterosteus aculeatus*	0.3 g	Static	20	25	96-h LC$_{50}$	1.5	Katz & Chadwick (1961)

[a] Static, static conditions (water unchanged for duration of test); flow, flow-through conditions; int. flow, intermittent flow-through conditions; endrin concentration in water maintained continuously

reduction in growth, and survival was reduced at 1.21 µg/litre; with a 72-h exposure, growth was reduced at 0.63 µg/litre, and all fish died at 1.15 µg/litre. Continuous exposure to 0.38 µg/litre for 30 days significantly reduced growth, and all fish died at 0.73 µg/litre (Jarvinen et al., 1988).

Sheephead minnows (*Cyprinodon variegatus*) were exposed continuously for 23 weeks to endrin from the embryonic stage through hatching, until adulthood and spawning. The average exposure concentrations were 0 (control), 0.027, 0.077, 0.12, 0.31, and 0.72 µg/litre. The resultant progeny were monitored to determine effects on their survival, growth, and reproduction. Embryos exposed to 0.31 and 0.72 µg/litre hatched early; all fry exposed to 0.72 µg/litre died by day 9 of exposure. At 0.31 µg/litre, fry were initially stunted and some died. Survivors seemed unaffected until maturity, when some females died during spawning; fewer eggs were fertile, and survival of exposed progeny was decreased. No significant effect was observed throughout the life cycle at an exposure concentration of 0.12 µg/litre (Hansen et al., 1977).

Endrin was tested in flagfish (*Jordanella floridae*) at 0.21, 0.29, and 0.39 µg/litre for 30 days. Only the highest concentration decreased survival, and the two highest dose levels affected the mean number of eggs produced (Hermanutz et al., 1985).

7.2.2.3 Studies of resistance

Populations of mosquito fish (*Gambusia affinis*) developed high levels of resistance to endrin and other cyclodiene insecticides as a result of inadvertent exposure to agricultural sprays. Susceptible fish (male) showed a LC_{50} of 8.3 mg/litre and resistant fish, 161 mg/litre. Genetic crossing studies show that endrin resistance is inherited as a single, autosomal, intermediate gene (Yarbrough et al., 1986).

Pesticide-susceptible and -resistant mosquito fish were exposed to ^{14}C-endrin at 20 or 1000 µg/litre, and liver and brain were assayed to determine any difference in distribution, uptake, and nerve binding patterns (Fabacher & Chambers, 1976). The results are summarized in Table 18. Endrin was taken up faster by brain and liver from susceptible fish than resistant fish. In resistant fish, at least at a high lethal concentration (1000 µg/litre), endrin entered the brain slowly and accumulated in the liver, suggesting a more efficient blood–brain barrier in resistant than in susceptible fish. Extraction studies provided some evidence that endrin binds more readily to nonessential protein complexes in the nervous tissue of resistant fish, consequently decreasing the amount of endrin available to produce a toxic effect.

Table 18. Mean quantities of endrin (in mg/kg tissue) in brain and liver of susceptible and resistant mosquito fish

Genotype	At 20 µg/litre			At 1000 µg/litre		
	Brain	Liver	Brain:liver	Brain	Liver	Brain:liver
Susceptible	16.98	33.28	0.51	149.31	160.27	0.93
Resistant	8.83	16.84	0.52	57.52	353.42	0.16
Susceptible: resistant	1.90	1.90	1.00	2.60	0.45	5.80

Cell membrane fractions from resistant mosquito fish bound more endrin than those from susceptible fish, and mitochondria from the liver of the resistant genotype bound less endrin than those from susceptible fish. Differences in endrin uptake, retention of endrin by brain cell membranes, a blood–brain barrier, and a structural difference in myelin may account for the resistance of some mosquito fish to endrin (Wells & Yarbrough, 1972).

In resistant and non-resistant populations of golden shiner (*Notemigonus crysoleucas*), blue gill sunfish (*Lepomis macrochirus*), and green sunfish (*Lepomis cyanellus*), the median tolerated limit at 36 h was 3.0, 1.5, and 3.4 µg/litre for non-resistant strains and 310, 300, and 160 µg/litre for resistant fish, respectively (Ferguson et al., 1964).

7.2.2.4 Interaction with other chemicals

The joint action of endrin with malathion on mortality in flagfish (*Jordanella floridae*) consisted of enhanced effects at concentrations that had no effect when the substances were tested individually. The effects of the mixture on growth followed a simple additive model. Malathion did not modify the effect of endrin on egg production. In a separate test, malathion did not affect the uptake or elimination of endrin (Hermanutz et al., 1985).

In a study of the interaction between the accumulation and elimination of ^{14}C-endrin and ^{14}C-DDT in mosquito fish (*Gambusia affinis*), fish about

Effects on organisms in the environment

4 cm long were exposed to a nominal concentration of 3.94 nM endrin or DDT, or to a mixture of the compounds. Prior exposure to DDT for 4 h generally reduced the accumulation of endrin in serum, gall-bladder, and whole bodies, whereas prior exposure to endrin for 4 h had little effect on DDT accumulation. Simultaneous exposure to DDT and endrin reduced the accumulation of DDT in the gall-bladder over the 4 h of exposure and in the whole bodies during the first hours, and it reduced the accumulation of endrin in gall-bladder and in the whole body. Endrin levels in fish exposed subsequently only to DDT or DDE were significantly higher in gall-bladder and were reduced in the whole body over 4 h. The interactions observed may be the result of competition for and/or displacement of insecticides from mutual binding sites (Denison et al., 1985).

In a study of the relative binding and competition between organochlorine pesticides for serum binding sites, incubation with serum from mosquito fish led to their association primarily with the vitellogenin/lipoprotein and albumin fractions. Preincubation of serum with endrin significantly reduced the quantity of ^{3}H-DDT that was bound subsequently, while the reverse was not observed. Although the reason for the apparent quantitative decrease in binding is unknown, this phenomenon may be of toxicological importance (Denison & Yarbrough, 1985).

7.2.2.5   Special studies

Fingerlings of carp (*Cyprinus carpio*) exposed to endrin at the LC_{50} (0.0065 mg/kg) for 24 h showed clear inhibition of α-amylase activity in the liver (Datta & Ghose, 1985).

A group of 240 rainbow trout (*Salmo gairdneri*) were exposed to endrin at 0.12–0.15 µg/litre for 30 days; one untreated and one solvent control group were used. On day 30, 10 fish from each group were sacrificed and examined for the ability of peritoneal macrophages to phagocytize latex beads. The remaining fish were immunized with 10 µg of *Yersinia ruckeri* O-antigen and exposure to endrin continued. Assays for migration inhibition factor, plaque forming cells, and serum agglutination titre were performed 2, 14, and 30 days after inoculation, and serum was collected from all fish to determine the cortisol concentration. Exposure to endrin had no effect on the phagocytic ability of peritoneal macrophages, but the responses in the three assays were significantly reduced in comparison with the control values. Serum cortisol concentrations were significantly elevated in the endrin-treated fish. The study did not, however, elucidate

Table 19. Acute toxicity of endrin to amphibians

Organism	Size/age	Static/flow[a]	Temp. (°C)	Hardness (mg CaCO$_3$/l)	pH	Parameter (mg/l)	Concentration (μg/l)	Reference
Bullfrog *Rana catesbiana*	2–5 g	Flow	18–23			96-h LC$_{50}$	2.5	Thurston et al. (1985)
Leopard frog *Rana spenocephala*	Eggs	Flow	20	100	7.2–7.5	24-h LC$_{50}$	2.5	Hall & Swineford (1980)
	Larvae	Flow	20	100	7.2–7.5	96-h LC$_{50}$	6	
	Subadult	Flow	20	100	7.2–7.5	96-h LC$_{50}$	5	
Frog *Rana hexadactyla*	0.5 g	Static	14	20	6.2	96-h LC$_{50}$	0.21	Khangarot et al. (1985)
Western chorus frog *Pseudacris triseriata*	Tadpole	Static	15	44	7.1	96-h LC$_{50}$	120	Mayer & Ellersieck (1986)
Fowlers toad *Bufo woodhousei fowleri*	Tadpole	Static	15	44	7.1	96-h LC$_{50}$	180	Mayer & Ellersieck (1986)

[a] Static, static conditions (water unchanged for duration of test); flow, flow-through conditions; endrin concentration in water maintained continuously

Effects on organisms in the environment

the mechanism of immune suppression, other than showing that a stress response had occurred (Bennett & Wolke, 1987a). In another study, therefore, control fish were fed cortisol at 20 mg/kg and metyrapone at 35 mg/kg body weight, and endrin-exposed fish received metyrapone at 35 mg/kg body weight per day in the diet. The fish that received cortisol had significantly reduced responses in all three assays; but in the endrin-exposed fish that received metyrapone, the migration inhibition factor response was completely restored, the plaque forming cell response was restored to 61%, and serum agglutination titres to 69%. These results indicate that elevated serum cortisol concentration plays a central role in repressing the immune response (Bennett & Wolke, 1987b).

The concentrations of serum glucose, liver and muscle glycogen, cortisol, protein, and cholesterol were determined in carp (*Cyprinus carpio*) exposed to endrin at 2 μg/litre for 6, 24, and 72 h. Only the concentration of cortisol in serum was clearly decreased (Gluth & Hanke, 1985).

7.2.3 Amphibia

The acute toxicity of endrin to amphibians is summarized in Table 19.

7.3 Terrestrial organisms

The acute oral toxicity of endrin for terrestrial animals is high. The available LD_{50} values are summarized in Table 20.

7.3.1 Honey bees

The 48-h LD_{50} of endrin in worker honey bees (*Apis mellifera*) using a dusting technique was 2.02 μg/bee (Atkins et al., 1973). The LD_{50} for bees after contact was 0.65 μg/bee, and the acute oral LD_{50} was 0.46 μg/bee (Oomen, 1986).

Table 20. Acute oral LD_{50}s of endrin for terrestrial species

Species	LD_{50} (mg/kg body weight)	Reference
Birds		
Mallard (*Anas platyrhynchos*)	5.6 (2.7–11.7)	Hudson et al. (1984)
Pigeon (*Columbia livia*)	2.0–5.0	
Pheasant (*Phasianus colchicus*)	1.8 (1.1–2.8)	
Sharp-tailed grouse (*Pedioecetes phasianellus*)	1.06 (0.552–2.04)	
California quail	1.19 (0.857–1.65)	
Redwinged blackbird (*Agelaius phoeniceus*)	2.37	Schafer et al. (1983)
Starling (*Sturnus vulgaris*)	2.37–3.16	
Quail (*Coturnix coturnix*)	4.22	
Mammals		
Big brown bat (*Eptesicus fuscus*)	5–8	Luckens & Davis (1965)
Pine mouse (*Microtus pitymys pinetorum*)	2.6/19.0 1.3/36.4 (susceptible/resistant)	Petrella et al. (1975) Webb et al. (1973)

7.3.2 Birds

7.3.2.1 Acute toxicity

The LD_{50}s of endrin for some bird species are given in Table 20.

7.3.2.2 Short-term toxicity

Groups of 40 one-day-old quail were fed endrin at dietary levels of 0, 0.5, 1, 5, 10, 20, or 50 mg/kg of diet. Survival was adversely affected in all test groups, and there were no survivors beyond two weeks among birds fed 10 mg/kg or more. Food consumption was abnormally low, and symptoms involved lack of muscular coordination, tremors, and occasional

Effects on organisms in the environment

convulsive movements. Similar results were obtained in 40 one-day-old pheasants fed endrin at dietary levels of 5 or 20 mg/kg, none of which survived beyond 8 days (Dewitt, 1965).

Groups of 20 seven-day-old chicks were unaffected by diets containing endrin at 0, 1.5, or 3 mg/kg. When the concentration was increased to 6 or 12 mg/kg, the birds became highly excitable and failed to gain weight in comparison with controls. The survival rates over a 12-week period were 85 and 5%, respectively, compared with 100% in the controls (Sherman & Rosenberg, 1954).

The LC_{50} values for 2–3-week-old bobwhite quail (*Colinus virginianus*), Japanese quail (*Coturnix coturnix japonica*), ring-necked pheasants (*Phasianus colchicus*), and mallards (*Anas platyrhynchos*) (8–13 birds per group) fed endrin in their diet for 5 days followed by 3 days of untreated diet, were 14–22 mg/kg diet (Hill et al., 1975; Hill & Camardese, 1986).

7.3.2.3 Studies of reproduction

In a study of reproduction in pheasants, a diet containing endrin at 10 mg/kg reduced egg production and chick survival; diets containing up to 2 mg/kg did not affect egg production, fertility, hatchability, or chick survival (Dewitt, 1965).

Groups of five female and two male mallard ducks (*Anas platyrhynchos*) were administered diets containing endrin at 0, 0.5, or 3.0 mg/kg for a 12-week oviposition period. Egg production was not affected. The eggs were incubated, and infertile eggs, embryo survival, and hatchability were measured. Fertility and hatchability were not affected, although a 9.6% drop in embryo survival was observed in the group that had received the highest dose. Endrin residues in body fat were 3.4 mg/kg of tissue in the group that received 0.5 mg/kg and 19.3 mg/kg in the group that received 3.0 mg/kg. The concentrations were higher in females than in males. The endrin residue levels in eggs were none detected in the controls, 0.43 mg/kg in the group fed 0.5 mg/kg, and 2.75 mg/kg in the group fed 3.0 mg/kg (Roylance et al., 1985).

Three groups of 27 pairs of mallards were fed endrin at 0, 1, or 3 mg/kg of dry duck mash from December to the summer to investigate the influence on reproduction and health. Birds fed 1 mg/kg reproduced as well as the controls; they had significantly greater success in hatching fertile eggs than did those fed 0 or 3 mg/kg and their clutches hatched earlier (not significantly) than those of birds fed 3 mg/kg. Endrin accumulated in eggs to a mean level of 1.1 mg/kg (wet weight) in the group fed 1 mg/kg and 2.9 mg/kg in the group fed 3 mg/kg. The concentration of endrin in adipose tissue was four to seven times higher than that in eggs (Spann et al., 1986).

7.3.2.4 Interaction with other chemicals

The toxicity of combinations of chlordane and endrin was studied in 14-week-old male and female bobwhite quail. Eight birds received 10 mg/kg chlordane in the diet for 10 weeks; 20 quail were treated with 10 mg/kg chlordane for 10 weeks followed immediately by 10 mg/kg endrin (98%) in the diet; a fourth group of 20 birds received only 10 mg/kg endrin in the diet. The pesticides were dissolved in propylene glycol. After 9–10 days on a control diet, survivors were sacrificed and their brains dissected. No deaths occurred among the birds fed the control diet or 10 mg/kg chlordane. With endrin alone, 15 birds died, and with the combination 14 birds died. In birds that received endrin alone, the residue levels in the brain were 0.34–1.84 mg/kg in those that died and 0.28–0.62 mg/kg in the survivors. In the birds fed chlordane and endrin, the residue levels were 0.17–1.25 mg/kg in birds that died and 0.14–0.56 mg/kg in survivors. Birds treated with the combination had considerably more chlordane residues in their brains than did those fed chlordane alone. The main conclusion of this study was that the additive toxicity of closely related chemicals should be taken into account in diagnosing cause of death (Ludke, 1976).

7.3.2.5 Special studies

The influence of endrin at 5 and 10 mg/kg of feed on the activity of various enzymes in the serum of juvenile cockerels was studied. The greatest increases in activity were measured for glutamate oxalacetate transaminase, cholinesterase, and alkaline phosphatase. Smaller increases were observed for creatine kinase, glutamate dehydrogenase, α-hydroxybutyrate dehydrogenase, and phosphohexose isomerase (Horn et al., 1987).

Effects on organisms in the environment

7.3.2.6 Behavioural studies

The effect of a sub-lethal dose of endrin (2 mg/kg diet) on avoidance responses was studied in eight pens of 25 seven-day-old Coturnix quail chicks for 14 days. The stimulus used to elicit avoidance was a moving silhouette, and the response was measured daily. Group avoidance response was significantly suppressed by exposure to endrin, but the behaviour returned to normal after 2 days on untreated diet (Kreitzer & Heinz, 1974).

Adult male bobwhite quail (*Colinus virginianus*) were fed a diet containing endrin at 0.1 or 1.0 mg/kg for 138 days (beginning at 3 days of age), and then their performance in five non-spatial discrimination reversal tasks was studied. Treated birds made 36–139% more errors than controls, and birds fed the lower dose made significantly more errors than those given the higher dose after reversal 3 or 4 in the first three tests. The effects of endrin were reversed after 50 days on untreated feed. The principal effect of endrin was to impair the birds' ability to solve a novel problem. The mean levels of endrin residues in the brain were 0.075 mg/kg wet weight in those given the lower dose and 0.35 mg/kg for those on the higher dose (Kreitzer, 1980).

7.3.3 Mammals

7.3.3.1 Toxicity

The LC_{50} values for short-tailed male and female shrews (*Blarina brevicauda*) aged 180, 105–150, and 30–75 days were 87–174 mg/kg diet for 14 days (Blus, 1978).

Five groups each of 13–14 pairs of Saskatchewan deer mice (*Peromyscus maniculatus*) of various ages were fed endrin at 0, 1, 2, 4, or 7 mg/kg of diet for intermittent periods, between which the animals were either fed a normal diet or were subjected to 48-h starvation. The animals were sacrificed by exposing them to cold stress at −16 °C and the time of death recorded. No influence was found on litter production, frequency, or mean litter size. At the higher levels of feeding, postnatal mortality before weaning was increased. Significant parental mortality occurred at 4 mg/kg and higher and appeared to be dose-dependent (Morris, 1968). (Remark: Since the animals in this study were captured in the field and the periods of feeding alternated with short periods of starvation in an effort to simulate possible conditions in the field, this study is of only limited value).

The effects of endrin at 8.0 oz/acre (0.56 kg/ha) on unenclosed field populations of meadow voles (*Microtus pennsylvanicus*) and deer mice (*Peromyscus maniculatus*) were investigated in 1966–68. Animals were trapped live on adjacent 7-acre (2.8 ha) plots each summer at regular intervals, before and after a single application of endrin. Immediate, significant declines in the number of voles were seen on the experimental plot, but no long-term toxicological effects were observed. The population rapidly recovered, exceeding the initial and control numbers in all three years. The experimental vole population thus appears to have responded to endrin as it would to a local depopulation by trapping. The mouse population decreased significantly after the application of endrin in 1966 and did not recover, and the highly unstable, transitory population on the experimental plot indicated a long-term toxicological effect (Morris, 1970, 1972).

7.3.3.2 Studies of resistance

^{14}C-Endrin in corn oil was administered to a resistant and a susceptible strain of pine mice (*Microtus pitymus pinetorum*) orally at 0.5 mg/kg body weight, as follows: days 1–5, unlabelled endrin; days 6–14, ^{14}C-endrin; and day 15 unlabelled endrin. Total recovery of ^{14}C in both faeces and urine was 76% for the resistant strain and 53% for the susceptible strain. The two strains produced the same major faecal and urine metabolite, but the resistant strain produced about twice the quantity as the susceptible strain. The quantitative differences in the excretion of more polar endrin metabolites may indicate metabolic differences between the two strains and, consequently, the greater tolerance of the resistant strain to toxic effects (Petrella et al., 1975). The major metabolite was identified as *anti*-12-hydroxyendrin; one of the other more polar metabolites, found in minor quantities, was suggested to be a tertiary alcohol of endrin (Petrella et al., 1977).

The degree of toxicity of endrin in first-generation progeny of susceptible and resistant strains and a cross of the two strains of pine mice was studied by Webb et al. (1973). The LD_{50} for offspring of susceptible × susceptible parentage was 5.0 mg/kg body weight; that for resistant × resistant, 21.1 mg/kg; and that for susceptible × resistant, 8.6 mg/kg. These results offer preliminary support for a genetic mechanism with intermediate dominance. An increase in resistance against the toxic effects of endrin was demonstrated in wild pine mice trapped in orchards where endrin had been used for years. The oral LD_{50} in susceptible mice was

Effects on organisms in the environment

about 3 mg/kg body weight and that in resistant mice, an average of 36 mg/kg body weight. The increased resistance appeared to be heritable in the first generation (Webb & Horsfall, 1967; Webb et al., 1973). Although differences in the rate of metabolism of endrin could be demonstrated, especially in the activity of mixed-function oxidase, these did not appear to be sufficiently large to explain the resistance (Hartgrove et al., 1977).

7.4 Effects in the field

Episodes have been reported in which endrin was concluded to be the cause of death in fish and birds. Numerous fish kills were reported from the sugar-cane growing areas of Louisiana in 1960–63. No association with variables such as dissolved oxygen, pH, or temperature was found, but following the development of sensitive analytical techniques it was concluded that the fish had been killed by endrin (Mount & Putnicki, 1966). Surface runoff from fields was reported to be the main source of the endrin that contaminated the rivers (Lauer et al., 1966), although effluent from an insecticide plant may have contributed since the fish contained two chemicals involved in endrin manufacture (Mount & Putnicki, 1966). Levels of endrin found in studies of fish in the wild are given in section 5.1.4.2.

Declines in the population of brown pelicans in Louisiana were attributed to endrin, although at least six other organochlorine pesticides and polychlorinated biphenyls were found in the animals (Blus et al., 1975; King et al., 1977). The eggs of brown pelicans (*Pelecanus occidentalis*) in Texas, USA, were examined for endrin residues in 1975–81. The compound was recovered only in 1975, in 15 of 18 eggs, at levels of 0.1–0.3 mg/kg. In the same year, the highest levels of endrin were found in pelican eggs in Louisiana, and this maximum coincided with the deaths of large numbers of brown and white pelicans (*P. erhyrorhyncos*) (King et al., 1985).

Endrin was found in one of ten eggs of the American white pelican (*Pelecanus erythrorhynchos*) collected in 1969, at 0.20 mg/kg, and in two of 35 samples collected in 1981, at up to 0.18 mg/kg wet weight. Brains of pelicans found dead in the period 1975-81 had levels up to 0.80 mg/kg. No endrin was found in eggs of the western grebe (*Aechmophorus accidentalis*) collected in 1981. It was concluded that endrin had caused some of the deaths among pelicans in California (Boellstorff et al., 1985).

The death of sandwich terns in The Netherlands was attributed to the discharge of a combination of endrin and related pesticides into an estuary from a manufacturing plant (Koeman et al., 1967, 1969; Koeman, 1971).

On several occasions in Victoria, Australia, large numbers of wild birds, in particular pigeons (*Columba livia*), sparrows (*Passer domesticus*) and Indian mynahs (*Gracula religiosa*), were observed to be paralysed or in convulsions (Reece et al., 1985). The crops and livers contained endrin at levels of up to 1.2 mg/kg.

Fulvous whistling ducks (*Dendrocygna bicolor*), which nest in rice fields along the south-eastern coast of Texas, USA, suffered a major decline in population in the late 1960s, which was attributed to exposure to dieldrin or aldrin. Organochlorine pesticides were determined in 1983 in the carcasses of 15 adult ducks immediately after their arrival in Texas from Mexico in the spring and before departure from Mexico in the autumn. Four of the ducks with high levels of dieldrin residues also had residues of endrin; and four other ducks, collected in 1967 and 1969, had endrin residues. The geometric mean levels in the different years were 0.03–0.08 mg/kg wet weight; in juveniles in 1960-69, the geometric mean level was 0.16 mg/kg (Flickinger et al., 1986).

The effects of endrin on wildlife were studied in 1981–83 in fruit orchards in Washington, USA. A single application of endrin after harvest resulted in acute and chronic toxicity to a variety of avian species; most deaths occurred soon after the application, but several raptors died during the spring and summer. The brains of 73 of 125 birds contained endrin at < 0.10–0.80 mg/kg; detectable levels occurred most frequently in the brains of galliforms and falconiforms. The species in which the greatest numbers of deaths attributed to endrin occurred include California quail (*Callipepla california*), chukars (*Alectoris chukar*), and common barn owls (*Tyto alba*). Of the 97 eggs analysed, 68 contained detectable endrin residues: 51 had levels of < 0.10 mg/kg, and the eggs of 10 species contained 0.01–0.17 mg/kg wet weight (range, none detected to 1.67). The authors concluded that endrin was toxic to wildlife, although there was no evidence that it affected reproductive success or population level (Blus et al., 1989).

Levels found in birds in the wild are also given in section 5.1.4.1.

7.5 Appraisal of effects on organisms in the environment

Use of endrin in agriculture is the major source of its presence in the environment, but discharge of waste material from manufacturing and formulating plants has contributed to local contamination. World-wide monitoring surveys have shown that the concentrations of endrin in the biosphere are generally very low (Table 10), both absolutely and relatively: The levels of residues of other organochlorine compounds, particularly DDE and polychlorinated biphenyls, are generally 100 times or higher than those of endrin.

Toxicologically significant levels of endrin residues have been found locally in fish and other organisms, particularly in cases in which endrin was applied near rivers and lakes and when runoff occurred into waterways. Residues may also occur when endrin is used as a seed dressing or in bait to control rodents.

The most serious adverse ecological effects that have been reported were the fish kills (and associated adverse effects on brown pelican populations) in the Mississippi River system in the USA. Although the initial evidence for ascribing these effects to endrin was circumstantial, the results of analyses of dead fish were considered to confirm a causal relationship; there is little doubt that endrin was a contributory factor in at least some of these fish kills. The evidence that endrin was the primary cause of the decline in the brown pelican population is less convincing, since the harmful effects on reproductive success have been attributed to DDE and other factors (Blus et al., 1974, 1979).

In summary, agricultural application of endrin should be such as to avoid or minimize contamination of waterways, either by overspraying or runoff or by leaching from dressed seed in rice-growing areas. The effects of the use of baits containing endrin for rodent control on non-target organisms should be assessed in the light of local circumstances. Finally, effluents from manufacturing and formulating plants must be treated adequately before being discharged into waterways.

8. EFFECTS ON EXPERIMENTAL ANIMALS AND *IN VITRO*

The toxicology and risk assessment of endrin have been reviewed (US EPA, 1987a,b; Anon., 1988a,b).

8.1 Acute toxicity of technical-grade endrin

8.1.1 Oral administration

Endrin is highly toxic when given by the oral route and is more acutely toxic to mammals than its stereoisomer dieldrin (WHO, 1989), with an acute oral LD_{50} of 7.5–17.8 mg/kg body weight (Table 21), compared with 50–60 mg/kg for dieldrin. There appears to be a sex-dependent sensitivity to the acute effects of endrin, female animals being more sensitive than males. A species-dependent sensitivity has also been reported, monkeys and cats being more susceptible than mice and rats.

Signs of intoxication may include increased irritability and tremor, followed by tonic–clonic convulsions, ataxia, dyspnoea, gasping, and cyanosis. Convulsions usually occur 30–60 min after an oral dose, and death may occur within 24 h after the administration of a lethal dose (Speck & Maaske, 1958). Animals that survive poisoning recover completely with no delayed or persistent effect.

8.1.2 Dermal administration

The acute dermal LD_{50}s for technical endrin in various animal species are given in Table 22. Endrin is highly toxic when applied as a solution in hydrocarbon solvents but moderately toxic when applied as a dry powder. The signs of poisoning are similar to those seen after oral administration.

8.1.3 Parenteral administration

The acute LD_{50}s for technical-grade endrin given by parenteral routes of administration are shown in Table 23.

Table 21. Oral LD_{50}s for technical-grade endrin

Species (age)	Vehicle	LD_{50} (mg/kg body weight)		Reference
		Males	Females	
Mouse	Corn oil	8.6	–	Spynu (1964)
Mouse	Unknown	13	13	Gray et al. (1981)
Rat (4–5 weeks)	Peanut oil	28.8	16.8	Treon et al. (1955)
Rat (6 months)	Peanut oil	43.4	7.3	Treon et al. (1955)
Rat (6 months)	Peanut oil	40.0	–	Speck & Maaske (1958)
Rat (adult)	Peanut oil	17.8	7.5	Gaines (1960)
Rat (7 weeks)	Cottonseed oil	27	–	Boyd & Stefec (1969)
Rat (12–14 weeks)	Dimethyl sulfoxide	5.6[a]	5.3[a]	Bedford et al. (1975b)
Rat (12–13 weeks)	Corn oil	8.9	4.0	Carter & Simpson (1978)
Rat	Corn oil	9.0	–	Spynu (1964)
Rat	Unknown	4	4	Gray et al. (1981)
Rabbit	Peanut oil	–	7–10	Treon et al. (1955)
Guinea-pig	Peanut oil	36.0	16.0	Treon et al. (1955)
Hamster (golden Syrian)	Corn oil	–	18.6	Chernoff et al. (1979)
Hamster (golden Syrian) (6 weeks)	Unknown	12	17.0	Cabral et al. (1979)
Hamster	Unknown	18	18	Gray et al. (1981)

Table 21. (contd)

Species (age)	Vehicle	LD$_{50}$ (mg/kg body weight)		Reference
		Males	Females	
		Lethal dose:		
Cat	Cod liver oil	3–6		Ressang et al. (1958); Cook & Casteel (1985); Casteel & Cook (1985)
Monkey (*Macacus mulatta*)	Peanut oil	3		Treon et al. (1955)
Monkey (*Macacus speciosa*)	Unknown	12		Barth (1967)
Domestic goat	Unknown		25–50	Tucker & Crabtree (1970)
Mule deer	Unknown		6.25–12.5	Hudson et al. (1984)

[a] Endrin of 99% purity

Table 22. Dermal LD_{50}s for technical-grade endrin

Species (age)	Vehicle	LD_{50} (mg/kg body weight)		Reference
		Males	Females	
Rat	Xylene	18	15	Gaines (1960, 1969)
Rat	Shellsol A	10–20	5–10	Carter & Simpson (1978)
Rat	Toluene	≈10	≈10	Carter & Simpson (1978)
Rat	Corn oil	12.5	–	Spynu (1964)
Rabbit	None	–	Minimum lethal dose: 60–94	Treon et al. (1955)
Cat	Cod-liver oil	Lethal dose: ≈150		Ressang et al. (1958)

Table 23. Parental LD_{50}s for technical-grade endrin

Species	Route	Vehicle	LD_{50} (mg/kg body weight)	Reference
Mouse	Intraperitoneal	Corn oil	5.6	Graves & Bradley (1965)
Mouse	Intravenous	Dimethyl sulfoxide	2.3	Walsh & Fink (1970, 1972)
Dog	Intravenous	Ethanol	3	Hinshaw et al. (1966)

8.1.4 Toxicity of metabolites and isomers

8.1.4.1 Mammalian metabolites

In a comparative study, the acute oral LD_{50}s of endrin and three of its metabolites were determined in rats (Table 24). When the brains of some of the rats were analysed for the presence of endrin and its metabolites, the concentration of 12-ketoendrin in male rats given endrin at 60 mg/kg body weight was found to be higher (mean, 0.3 mg/kg) than that of endrin (0.07 mg/kg) 22 h after dosing. In male rats intoxicated with syn-12-hydroxyendrin or 12-ketoendrin (at 16 mg/kg body weight each), the concentrations of 12-ketoendrin in the brain 30 min after dosing were much higher (mean values, 1.9 and 1.4 mg/kg, respectively) than those in the brains of rats given a similar but non-toxic dose of anti-12-hydroxyendrin (mean, 0.09 mg/kg) and killed at the same time. The signs of intoxication were similar to those of endrin (Bedford et al., 1975b).

Table 24. Acute oral toxicity of mammalian metabolites of endrin in rats

Compound	Oral LD_{50} (mg/kg body weight)			
	Male		Female	
	Mean	95% CI	Mean	95% CI
Endrin	5.6	3.0–7.9	5.3	3.6–7.4
anti-12-Hydroxyendrin	2.4	2.0–3.0	5.5	4.2–7.2
syn-12-Hydroxyendrin	1.2	0.6–1.7	2.8	0.8–4.0
12-Ketoendrin	1.1	0.7–1.5	0.8	0.5–1.2

[a]95% CI, 95% confidence interval

Effects on experimental animals and in vitro

These results suggest that 12-ketoendrin may be the acute toxicant in rats. The production of 12-ketoendrin varies greatly from one mammalian species to another, however, and none has been detected in birds of various species that were killed by endrin (Stickel et al., 1979).

8.1.4.2 Isomers

As described in section 4.2, endrin is changed under the influence of sunlight into delta-ketoendrin. The acute toxicity of this isomer is given in Table 25. It is less toxic than endrin, and, like endrin, it is more toxic to female than to male rats. The signs of intoxication are similar to those seen with endrin.

The acute tocixity of the endrin aldehyde has been reported to be > 500 mg/kg body weight in male mice (Phillips et al., 1962).

Table 25. Acute toxicity of delta-ketoendrin

Sex and species	Route	LD_{50} (mg/kg body weight)	Reference
Male rats	Oral	120–180	Soto & Deichmann (1967)
Female rats	Oral	10–36	
Male rats	Oral	62.1 (53.3–72.2)	Stanford Research Institute (1954)
Rats	Intravenous	5	Soto & Deichmann (1967)
Male rats	Intraperitoneal	82	Stanford Research Institute (1953)
Male mice	Oral	23.6 (19.9–28.0)	Stanford Research Institute (1954)
Male mice	Intraperitoneal	16.7	Stanford Research Institute (1953)

8.1.5 Acute toxicity of formulated material

8.1.5.1 Oral and dermal administration

Oral and dermal LD_{50} values for formulated endrin in rats (Muir, 1970) are presented in Table 26. Dry formulations were administered orally as 1–2% aqueous suspensions and dermally in both dry form and as 2–5% aqueous suspensions. In general, the type of formulation did not significantly alter the acute oral toxicity of endrin. The dermal toxicity of the 50% wettable powder was similar to that of the 20% emulsifiable concentrate; the 2% field strength dust was the least toxic.

Table 26. Oral and dermal LD_{50}s for endrin formulations in rats

Formulation	LD_{50} (mg/kg body weight)			
	Oral		Dermal	
	Formulation	Active material	Formulation	Active material
20% Emulsifiable concentrate	20	4.20	52.20 (undiluted)	10.90
50% Wettable powder	7.6	3.80	21.80 (dry) 14.40 (aqueous)	10.90 7.20
2% Field strength dust	275	5.50	5720 (dry) 1140 (aqueous)	114.40 22.80

From Muir (1970)

Ten rabbits (body weight, 2.4–4.1 kg) were treated with an emulsifiable concentrate containing 19.4% endrin on clipped skin at a dose of 200 mg/kg body weight, and the material was allowed to remain in contact with the skin for 24 h. Four of the 10 animals died within 48 h (Anderson et al., 1953). Two of 10 rabbits (body weight, 2.0–2.5 kg) treated similarly with a 25% dust concentrate died within 48 h (Hine et al., 1954).

8.1.5.2 Inhalation

Ten adult rats were exposed for 1 h to a mist of of an emulsifiable concentrate containing 19.4% by weight of endrin in xylene, at a

Effects on experimental animals and in vitro

concentration of endrin slightly exceeding 2000 mg/m^3 of air, and were observed for 48 h. The particle size of the mist and other details of exposure were not reported. Three of the animals died 1–14 h after exposure (Anderson et al., 1953).

Groups of 10 Long Evans rats were exposed for 1 h to 25% and 30% endrin dust concentrates at a concentration of 2000 mg/m^3 of air. Particle size and other details of exposure were not provided. Five rats exposed to the 30% and three exposed to the 25% dust died within 48 h after exposure (Hine et al., 1954).

8.2 Short-term exposure

8.2.1 Oral administration

8.2.1.1 Mouse

Feeding studies were conducted to estimate the maximum tolerated doses of endrin in B6C3F1 mice. Groups of five males and five females were given a normal diet or one containing endrin at 2.5–20 mg/kg for 6 weeks, followed by observation for another 2 weeks. Three males and four females given 10 mg/kg died, but no mortality occurred at 5 mg/kg. No data were provided on animals fed 20 mg/kg. Hyperexcitability was observed in male mice given doses > 5 mg/kg of diet. Mean body weight gains were comparable with those of controls. The maximum tolerated dose was calculated by extrapolation to be 5 mg/kg of diet (NCI, 1978, 1979).

8.2.1.2 Rat

Groups of three male and two to three female Carworth rats, either 29 days or 6 months old, received daily doses of endrin at 1, 2, or 5 mg/kg body weight in peanut oil by gavage, on five days per week for 67–72 days. All rats given 1 mg/kg survived; the increased mortality in the other groups was dose-related: 2/5 females at 2 mg/kg and 3/3 males at 5 mg/kg day died. Pathological findings at autopsy included diffuse degenerative changes in the liver, kidneys, and brain, while survivors showed no such changes. All treated animals lost weight and developed hypersensitivity to stimuli (Treon et al., 1955).

Groups of five male and five female adult Sprague-Dawley rats were given diets containing technical-grade endrin at 0, 1, 5, 25, 50, or 100 mg/kg diet over a maximal period of 16 weeks and were observed for behaviour, weight gain, feed consumption, mortality rate, and symptoms of toxicity. Alkaline phosphatase levels, determined once a week, were higher in rats fed endrin than in the control group, and the total average feed consumption of treated rats was less than that of the control group. All rats fed 100 mg/kg of diet died during the first two weeks of the study, and only two female rats fed 50 mg/kg of diet survived the experiment. All male rats given 1 mg/kg and all female rats given 1 and 5 mg/kg of diet survived. Males appeared to be more susceptible than females to endrin in this study. The symptoms of intoxication were hypersensitivity to stimuli and convulsions: hypersensitivity was noted in all rats, and convulsions occurred among rats receiving 25, 50, and 100 mg/kg diet. Weight loss was dose-dependent and significant in all rats treated with endrin (Nelson et al., 1956).

To estimate the maximum tolerated doses of endrin in Osborne-Mendel rats, groups of five males and five females were given diets with or without endrin for 6 weeks, followed by observation for another 2 weeks. Endrin was added to the diet in two-fold increasing concentrations of 2.5–80 mg/kg. Mortality was not increased at 10 mg/kg, and mean body weight gain was no different from that in controls. At 20 mg/kg of diet, one animal of each sex died. The maximum tolerated dose was calculated by extrapolation to be 15 mg/kg diet (NCI, 1978, 1979).

8.2.1.3 Rabbit

Four of five female rabbits given an oral dose of endrin at 1 mg/kg body weight on five days per week died following the administration of 2, 30, 35, and 50 doses, respectively. The fifth rabbit survived 50 doses over a period of 10 weeks. Diffuse degenerative changes were observed in the liver and kidneys but not in the brain (Treon et al., 1955).

8.2.1.4 Dog

Dogs (mainly two per group) fed endrin at 5–50 mg/kg of diet died within 50 days. They regurgitated their food, became lethargic, salivated, and later refused to eat; they became emaciated and developed respiratory distress and signs of stimulation of the central nervous system. Diffuse degenerative lesions in the brain, heart, liver, and kidneys, together with

Effects on experimental animals and in vitro

pulmonary hyperaemia and oedema were observed. Three dogs fed diets containing 4 mg/kg of diet for 6 months survived, but they showed reduced body weight gain and a slight increase in liver:body weight ratio; no histopathological change was observed. At 3 mg/kg of diet or less, growth was normal (Treon et al., 1955).

Beagles (one male and one female/group; control group, only one dog) were fed diets containing endrin at 0, 1, or 3 mg/kg for 80 weeks. No sign of intoxication was observed, and the weight gain of treated animals was comparable to that of controls. The ratios of kidney and heart to body weight were increased at 3 mg but not at 1 mg (about 0.045 mg/kg body weight). No histopathological change was found in the viscera (Treon et al., 1955).

Groups of three male and three female pure-bred beagle dogs (4–6 months old) were fed endrin in the diet at 0, 0.1, 0.5, 1, 2, or 4 mg/kg for two years. Additional groups of four male and four female dogs were fed endrin at 0, 1, or 4 mg/kg of diet. Two males and two females of each group were killed after 6 and 12 months of feeding; no other death occurred during the study. Convulsions were observed in three dogs at 4 mg and in one female at 2 mg; no other sign of intoxication or illness was apparent during the study. No adverse effect was noted on growth, food consumption, haematology, or urinalysis, and no compound-related change was found in serum alkaline phosphatase, prothrombin time, or any of the other clinical chemical parameters measured at regular intervals. All organ weights, relative as well as absolute, were normal, except for occasional, slight increases in liver weight in some of the females at 2 and 4 mg in the diet. The only histopathological change found was a slight to moderate vacuolation of liver cells in dogs fed 2 and 4 mg in the diet. No renal change was observed in any of the dogs (Jolley et al., 1969).

8.2.1.5 Domestic animals

Sheep and cattle fed diets containing endrin at 2.5 or 5 mg/kg for 112 days showed no indication of harmful effects (details not given) (Radeleff, 1956). The convulsions and muscular tremors that were induced in six 10–18-month-old male buffalo calves administered a 20% emulsion of endrin led to a significant rise in lactic acid concentration in the blood of the animals, possibly due to excessive production of the acid inside the fasciculating muscles (Verma et al., 1970).

8.2.2 Inhalation

Three mice, three rats, two guinea-pigs, two hamsters, four rabbits, and one cat were exposed to sublimed endrin vapour at an actual concentration of 5.44 mg/m^3 for 7 h/day on 5 days/week for up to 26 weeks. Two rabbits died after 26 and 90 exposures, respectively, and one mouse died after 22 exposures. No convulsions were observed, and all other animals survived. Surviving rabbits showed a granulomatous type of pneumonitis; no histological change was found in the other surviving animals (Treon et al., 1955).

8.2.3 Dermal administration

Three female rabbits with intact skin died after 19, 19, and 25 applications, respectively, of endrin as a dry powder at 150 m/kg body weight for 2 h/day on 5 days/week. Applications of 75 mg/kg resulted in the death of one of three rabbits after 8 weeks; the other two survived for 13–14 weeks—the end of exposure. Convulsions, tremors, and twitching of the facial muscles were the main signs of intoxication. Two of five rabbits (dose not specified) showed severe fatty degeneration of the liver (Treon et al., 1955).

8.3 Skin irritation

Dry powdered endrin was applied repeatedly at a dose of 75 or 150 mg/kg body weight for 2 h/day, 5 days/week for up to 14 weeks on intact or abraded skin of female rabbits (see section 8.2.3). No skin irritation was observed. Single applications of endrin as dry powder at doses up to 250 mg/kg body weight for 24 h on rabbit skin caused no gross or microscopic damage to the skin of the animals (Treon et al., 1955).

8.4 Reproduction, embryotoxicity, and teratogenicity

8.4.1 Reproduction

8.4.1.1 Mouse

CFW mice (20 males and 20 females) were fed diets containing endrin (96%) at 0 and 5 mg/kg for 120 days, beginning 30 days before mating.

Effects on experimental animals and in vitro

Significant parental mortality (32%) and reduced litter size were observed, but fertility, fecundity, and the number of litters produced per pair were not affected (Good & Ware, 1969).

8.4.1.2 Rat

Forty male and 80 female Long-Evans rats were fed endrin in the diet at 0, 0.1, 1, or 3 mg/kg over three generations, each generation breeding once. No difference in appearance, behaviour, body weight, or number or size of litters was seen. The weights of the liver, kidneys, and brain were normal, and no histopathological abnormality was seen in third-generation weanlings. The only significant effect was increased mortality of pups in the second and third generations of rats fed 3 mg/kg (Hine, 1965).

Ten male and 20 female Long-Evans rats were treated similarly, but each generation bred twice. Weanling rats were mated after 79 days on the diets (when they were 100 days old). All pups from the first litters were discarded at weaning, and the parent rats were mated again. Randomly selected pups from the second litters were maintained on the diets and mated when 100 days old; this was done for three generations. The number of pups in each litter was counted on the day of birth and on the fifth day; on the twenty-first day, the weanlings were counted and weighed and either sacrificed or saved for continuation. Parent rats were weighed, sacrificed, and examined grossly when no longer needed. Ten male and 10 female F_{3b} weanlings each from the controls and the highest dose-level group and five males and five females from the 0.1 and 1.0 mg groups were autopsied. Body, liver, kidney, and brain weights were recorded, and sections of these organs and from heart, lung, spleen, and testis were studied histologically. Appearance, behaviour, body weight, number and size of litters, organ weights, and histopathological appearance of F_{3b} weanlings were comparable with those in control animals. No effect on reproduction was observed in rats fed diets containing endrin at 2 mg/kg over three generations (Hine, 1968).

8.4.2 Embryotoxicity and teratogenicity

8.4.2.1 Mouse

Groups of 10 CD-1 mice were given a single oral dose of endrin (99%) at 2.5 mg/kg body weight (stated to be half the LD_{50}) in corn oil by gavage on day 9 of gestation; an untreated and a vehicle control group were also used. Fetuses were examined on day 18. No significant effect was observed on intrauterine death or fetal weight, but the incidence of total anomalies was increased over that in controls: 2/117 fetuses had cleft palates, three had open eye, and two had other anomalies. No data on maternal toxicity were reported (Ottolenghi et al., 1974).

These results could not be repeated by Kavlock et al. Female CD-1 mice were given endrin (99%) at 0 (vehicle), 0.5, or 1.0 (groups of 40 mice), or 1.5 or 2.0 mg/kg body weight (groups of 20 mice) in corn oil by gavage on days 7–17 of gestation. The animals were killed on day 18. Maternal deaths occurred in the 1.5 and 2 mg/kg groups, reduced maternal weight gain was observed at and above 1 mg/kg, and maternal liver weight was increased at 0.5 mg/kg and higher. Fetal weight and skeletal, and visceral maturity were adversely affected at doses of 1 mg/kg and above. No teratogenic effect or embryonic lethality was observed, even at doses that caused maternal death (Kavlock et al., 1981, 1987).

In a study of the effects of acute alterations in maternal health status upon fetal development in the mouse, groups of 21 or 40 pregnant CD-1 mice were given a single oral dose of technical-grade endrin at 0 (vehicle), 7 or 9 mg/kg body weight in corn oil on day 8 of gestation. The animals were killed on day 18 of gestation. Three of 21 animals given 7 mg/kg (14%) and 19/40 mice gievn 9 mg/kg (47%) died. Maternal weight gain was decreased in both test groups; the total number of implantation sites and number of viable litters were not affected, but fetal weight was reduced. Delays in ossification of the skeleton and an increased incidence of supernumary lumbar ribs were observed. Although three fetuses from one litter in the 9 mg/kg group had fused ribs, no significant increase in the incidence of malformations was found. A statistically significant, linear, inverse relationship between maternal weight gain and the presence of supernumary ribs in their offspring was found (Kavlock et al., 1985).

8.4.2.2 Rat

Five groups of 25 female CD rats were administered endrin (97%) in methocel in oral doses of 0, 0.1, 0.5, or 2 mg/kg body weight per day on days 6–15 of gestation, or vitamin A, used as a positive control. The animals were killed on day 20. The largest dose of endrin caused maternal toxicity, as evidenced by weight loss and mortality (two animals). The fetuses showed some slight growth retardation (not significant) but no increase in intrauterine death rate. No effect attributable to endrin was seen on the mean number of viable fetuses, post-implantation losses, implantations, corpora lutea, fetal sex ratio, or fetal external, soft-tissue, or skeletal abnormalities. Bent ribs were observed in 6/522 fetuses treated with endrin, but not in relation to dose. An increase in delayed ossification in sternebrae and skull of fetuses was seen in the treated groups in comparison with the untreated control group. Animals given vitamin A had a significantly increased number of post-implantation losses and malformed fetuses (Goldentahl, 1978a).

Groups of 32, 15, 28, 30, and 15 female CD rats were given oral doses of endrin (99%) in corn oil at 0, 0.075, 0.15, 0.30, or 0.45 mg/kg body weight on days 7–20 of gestation. Rats were killed on day 21. Maternal weight gain was reduced at dose levels above 0.15 mg/kg, but no increase in maternal liver weight was found. Fetal mortality, weight, degree of skeletal and visceral maturation, and incidences of skeletal and visceral anomalies showed no dose-related effect (Kavlock et al., 1981).

8.4.2.3 Hamster

Three groups of golden Syrian hamsters (7, 24, and 8 animals/group) received a single oral dose of endrin (99%) in corn oil at 5 mg/kg body weight (stated to be half the LD_{50}) on day 7, 8, and 9 of gestation, respectively. Two control groups were used, consisting of 57 untreated and 41 vehicle controls. The animals were killed on day 14. The number of resorptions and of dead fetuses was increased after treatment on days 7 or 8 and to a lesser extent in the vehicle controls. The live fetuses in all three treated groups showed significant growth retardation when compared with controls. The incidence of anomalies was high only after treatment on day 8: congenital abnormalities were seen in 28% of fetuses, with open eye in 22%, webbed foot in 16%, cleft palate in 5%, and fused ribs in 8%. The anomalies that appeared to be increased significantly but to almost the same extent at all three stages were fused ribs and cleft palate (Ottolenghi et al., 1974).

These results could not be repeated by other workers. Groups of 27–29 golden Syrian hamsters were administered oral doses of endrin (97%) in methocel at 0 (two control groups), 0.1, 0.75, or 2.5 mg/kg body weight on days 4–13 of gestation. The animals were killed on day 14. Body weight gains of the animals given 2.5 mg/kg were slightly reduced. Maternal appearance, behaviour, and survival, mean number of viable fetuses, post-implantation losses, implantations, corpora lutea, fetal body weight, and crown–rump length showed no change attributable to treatment.

The number of malformations in fetuses was not increased, but ossification of the sternebrae and certain ribs was delayed (Goldentahl, 1978b).

Groups of 18–87 golden Syrian hamsters (LVG strain) were given endrin (98%) as a solution in corn oil by gavage either as a single dose of 0.5, 1.5, 5, 7.5, or 10 mg/kg body weight on day 8 of pregnancy or as multiple daily doses of 0.75, 1.5, 2.5, or 3.5 mg/kg body weight on days 5–14 of pregnancy. All animals were killed on day 15. With single doses, no effect was found on maternal survival, pregnancy rate, weight change or liver:body weight ratio. The only sign of maternal toxicity was the occurrence of transient convulsions 2 h after dosing in one hamster given 10 mg. No compound-related difference was noted in the number of implantation sites, fetal death rate, or fetal weight; indicators of skeletal maturity were not affected. A dose-related increase in the incidence of fused ribs was found in the groups given 7.5 and 10 mg/kg; increased incidences of meningo-encephaloceles were observed at 5 mg/kg and above, with no dose–response relationship. No other compound-related skeletal or visceral anomaly was noted. In the study of multiple doses, maternal toxicity (reduced weight gain and increased mortality) and fetal toxicity (increased mortality, reduced weight, reduced skeletal ossification, and an increased percentage of irregular supra-occipitalis) were observed at doses of 1.5 mg/kg and higher. No treatment-related maternal or fetal effect occurred at 0.75 mg/kg per day (Chernoff et al., 1979).

8.4.2.4 Perinatal behavioural development

Rats exposed perinatally to endrin at 0, 0.075, 0.15, or 0.3 mg/kg body weight from gestation day 7 through day 15 of lactation showed no mortality and no influence on survival or growth. Pups of mothers exposed to 0.15 or 0.3 mg were more active than those of mothers exposed to 0.075 mg or those in the control group. No clear difference in ambulation was noted, and at 90 days of age there was no difference (Gray et al., 1981; Kavlock et al., 1987).

Golden Syrian hamsters (LVG strain) given endrin (98%) at 0 or 1.5 mg/kg body weight per day by gastric intubation on days 5–14 of gestation had a persistent increase in locomotor activity. Offspring of treated hamsters ambulated more than the controls in the open field at 15 days, and long-term observation of activity in the figure-8 maze indicated that a significant increase in this behaviour was still present at 125 days of age. Other behaviour patterns, including sexual, rearing and

Effects on experimental animals and in vitro

running, and wheel behaviour, were unaffected. Dams repeatedly exposed to endrin at 0.75 and 1.5 mg/kg body weight were markedly hypoactive under the same testing conditions in which the pups were hyperactive. The dose of 1.5 mg/kg body weight killed more than half of the dams (Gray et al., 1981; Kavlock et al., 1987).

8.4.3 Appraisal of reproductive effects

Endrin had no reproductive effects in three generations of rats at a level of 2 mg/kg of diet, equivalent to 0.1 mg/kg body weight. It had no teratogenic effect in mice, rats, or hamsters after oral exposure during the period of organogenesis. The significance of the anomalies observed in mice and hamsters by Ottolenghi et al. (1974) is uncertain. Studies in the same strain of the same species using more rigorous protocols and larger numbers of animals could not confirm their findings.

The lowest-observed-adverse-effect level for maternal toxicity was 1.0 mg/kg body weight in mice, 0.3 mg/kg body weight in rats, and 1.5 mg/kg body weight in hamsters. Embryotoxicity was observed at doses of 1 mg/kg body weight in mice and 1.5 mg/kg body weight in hamsters. The overall no-observed-adverse-effect levels in mice, rats, and hamsters were 0.5, 0.15, and 0.75 mg/kg body weight, respectively (Table 27).

8.5 Mutagenicity and related end-points

8.5.1 Effects on microorganisms

Endrin was not mutagenic in numerous studies using *Salmonella typhimurium* (TA98, TA100, TA1535, TA1537, TA1538, TA1950, TA1978, SL4525, SL4700), *Escherichia coli* (WP2 *uvr*A, WP2 *uvr*⁻, Gal R^S, WP2, *hcr*, p3478, W3100), K-12 (Pol A_1^+/Pol$_1^-$), WP67, CM611, and CM571 *Bacillus subtilis* (M45), *Saccharomyces cerevisiae* (D3, D7), and *Serratia marcescens* (a21, a742), with or without metabolic activation by rat or mouse liver S9 (Fahrig, 1974; Van Dijck & van de Voorde, 1976; Ercegovich & Rashid, 1977; Simmon et al., 1977; Nishimura et al., 1982; Waters et al., 1982; Glatt et al., 1983; Moriya et al., 1983; Rashid & Mumma, 1986).

Table 27. Teratogenicity and effects on reproduction of oral administration of endrin

Animal (strain)	Exposure period	NOAEL	LOAEL	Reference
Rat (Long Evans)	3 generations, 1 litter	1 mg/kg diet (0.05 mg/kg bw)	3 mg/kg diet (0.15 mg/kg bw): increased mortality of pups in F_2 and F_3 generations	Hine (1965)
Rat (Long Evans)	3 generations, 2 litters	2 mg/kg diet (0.1 mg/kg bw)		Hine (1968)
Mice (CD-1)	Days 7-17 of gestation	0.5 mg/kg bw	1 mg/kg bw: maternal and fetal weight, skeletal and visceral maturity	Kavlock et al. (1981, 1987)
Rat (CD)	Days 7-20 of gestation	0.15 mg/kg bw	0.30 mg/kg bw: reduced maternal weight gain	Kavlock et al. (1981)
Rat (CD)	Days 6-15 of gestation	0.5 mg/kg bw	2 mg/kg bw: maternal toxicity	Goldentahll (1978a)
Hamster	Days 5-14 of gestation	0.75 mg/kg bw	1.5 mg/kg bw: maternal and fetal toxicity	Chernoff et al. (1979)

Effects on experimental animals and in vitro

No mutagenic effect was observed in *S. typhimurium* strains TA98, TA100, TA1535, or TA1537, with and without metabolic activation with S9 from livers of Aroclor 1254-induced rats and hamsters in the presence of five concentrations of endrin (0–10 000 µg/plate) (Zeiger, 1987; Zeiger et al., 1987). No mutagenic effect was observed in *S. typhimurium* strains TA97, TA98, TA100, or TA102 with and without metabolic activation with Aroclor 1254-induced rat liver microsome fraction in the presence of seven concentrations of endrin (99.0%), from 1 ng/plate up to 1 mg/plate (Mersch-Sundermann et al., 1988).

8.5.2 Point mutations in mammalian cells

Endrin was weakly mutagenic in 6-thioguanine-resistant mouse FM3A cells (Morita & Umeda, 1984; abstract only).

8.5.3 Dominant lethal mutations

Endrin did not show detectable dominant lethality when given as a single intraperitoneal dose (0.76 or 3.8 mg/kg body weight) or daily oral doses (0.1 or 0.25 mg/kg body weight) for 5 days to seven or nine male ICR/Ha Swiss mice, respectively. This study involved a sequential mating procedure, in which one male was housed with three females for one week, repeated for 8 weeks (Epstein et al., 1972).

8.5.4 Chromosomal and cytogenetic effects

Endrin at 10^{-5} and 10^{-4} M, but not at 10^{-6}, produced a dose-related increase in the percentage of M1 metaphases and a dose-related decrease in that of M3 metaphases at 48 h in treated LAZ-007 human lympoid cells. This effect is closely related to the reduced rate of cell proliferation induced by endrin (Sobti et al., 1983).

Intratesticular injection of 0.25 mg endrin in saline to three albino rats doubled the percentage of chromosomal changes in comparison with that in the single control when the testes were studied histologically 10 days after the injection. Changes were scored in 70–75 cells/animal (Dikshith & Datta, 1973). The use of a single dose does not aid interpretation, and the increase in chromosomal abnormalities may be related to cytotoxicity rather than to a genetic effect. The relevance of this type of study in mutagenicity testing is unknown.

Chromosomal studies were carried out on lymphocytes from eight male workers exposed to endrin and from six unexposed workers from the same work area. No increase in the frequency of chromosomal abnormalities was found, whether taken individually or collectively (Dean, 1977).

Chromosomal aberrations were found in meiotic cells of barley and somatic cells of barley and *Vicia faba* grown from endrin-treated seeds (Wuu & Grant, 1966, 1967a,b). After treatment of root tips with 0.1% endrin (EC20 solution) for 1.5–2 h at 10 °C, the function of the spindle was destroyed and did not interfere with the spreading of the chromosomes during squash preparation. The centromeric region became distinct and visible in prophase–metaphase chromosomes. At higher concentrations contraction, stickiness, and fragmentation of chromosomes were seen (Bhowmik, 1978).

8.5.5 Host-mediated effects

In two studies, male CF1 mice were given single oral doses of endrin in dimethyl sulfoxide at 3.75 or 7.5 mg/kg body weight. Control mice were dosed with the solvent, and positive control groups were given a single oral dose of ethylmethanesulfonate at 400 mg/kg body weight. *Saccharomyces cerevisiae* JD1 suspensions were then injected intraperitoneally into each mouse, and the suspensions of *S. cerevisiae* were harvested and analysed after 5 h. No increase in mitotic gene conversion was detected (Brooks, 1976).

8.5.6 Sister chromatid exchange

Endrin at concentrations of 10^{-6}–10^{-4} mol/litre in dimethyl sulfoxide (the latter dose was a cytotoxic concentration) failed to increase the frequency of sister chromatid exchange significantly over the control value in rat liver microsomal S9-activated and unactivated incubation experiments using human lymphoid cells of the LAZ-007 cell line (Sobti et al., 1983).

8.5.7 Effects in Drosophila melanogaster

Endrin was not mutagenic to *Drosophila melanogaster* after injection at 0.2 μlitre of a 0.001% aqueous solution, in the Muller-5 test for recessive lethal mutations on the X-chromosome (Benes & Sram, 1969).

Effects on experimental animals and in vitro

8.5.8 Effects on DNA

Endrin at 10^{-3} or 3×10^{-3} mol/litre did not induce mutation in the adult rat liver epithelial culture/hypoxanthineguanine phosphoribosyl transferase assay (Williams, 1979).

DNA repair was not elicited in primary cultures of hepatocytes from CD-1 mice, Fischer 344 rats, or Syrian hamsters exposed to endrin for 18 h together with tritium-labelled thymine deoxyribonucleotide for incorporation during repair synthesis. DNA repair was measured autoradiographically. In rat and hamster liver cell cultures, a concentration of 10^{-3} mol/litre and in mouse liver cell cultures, 10^{-4} mol/litre endrin was tested (Maslansky & Williams, 1981).

Endrin did not induce unscheduled DNA synthesis in human lung fibroblast cells with or without metabolic activation by rat liver microsomes (five concentrations were tested, but they were not given in the paper) (Waters et al., 1982).

Endrin at eight concentrations ranging from 0.5 up to 1000 nmol/ml did not induce unscheduled DNA synthesis in primary rat hepatocytes or in a modified Ames test utilizing concentration gradient plates and 10 bacterial tester strains (eight *S. typhimurium* and two *E. coli*) (Probst et al., 1981)

8.5.9 Appraisal of mutagenicity and related end-points

Garrett et al. (1986) evaluated the activity of endrin in a series of tests: for reverse mutation (point/gene mutations in prokaryotes), forward mutation (point/gene mutations in eukaryotes), differential toxicity (primary DNA damage in prokaryotes), enhanced mitotic recombination, gene conversion and crossing-over, unscheduled DNA synthesis (primary DNA damage in eukaryotes), sister chromatid exchange, chromosomal breakage, and dominant lethality (chromosomal effects). Endrin gave negative results in all these tests.

The vast majority of the data indicate that endrin is not genotoxic; however, many of the studies would not reach current standards, or they give insufficient data to allow an independent assessment.

8.6   Long-term exposure

Groups of 20 male and 20 female Carworth rats (28 days old) were given diets containing endrin at 0, 1, 5, 25, 50, or 100 mg/kg. With 100 mg, two males and one female survived for 2 years; with 50 mg, four males but no female survived; and with 25 mg, 11 males and 5 females survived. Survival at the lower concentrations was comparable to that of the control group. Males appeared to be less susceptible than females to the toxic action of endrin. Signs of intoxication, hypersensitivity to external stimuli, and occasional convulsions were observed only at the two highest levels. The weight gain of females fed 1, 5, or 25 mg/kg of diet was equal to or greater than that of the controls after 40 weeks of feeding. In males fed 5 mg, growth retardation occurred during the first 20 weeks only, while males that received 25 mg showed significant reduction in body weight gain. The body weight gain of males fed 1 mg was comparable to that of controls. The liver:body weight ratios were increased in males fed 5 mg or more and in females fed diets with 25 mg or more. Histopathological examination of animals that died during exposure to the three higher dietary levels revealed diffuse degeneration of the liver, kidneys, brain, and adrenal glands. The few survivors at 50 and 100 mg showed degenerative changes in the liver only. No histopathological change was found in surviving rats fed 1, 5, or 25 mg/kg diet. There was no increase in the incidence of neoplasia in the treated groups compared to the control group (Treon et al., 1955).

This study indicates a no-effect level for endrin of 1 mg/kg of diet (about 0.05 mg/kg body weight) but is inadequate in several respects, e.g., survival rate, details of pathology, and haematological and clinical chemical data are not reported.

8.7   Carcinogenicity

8.7.1   Oral administration

8.7.1.1   Mouse

Groups of 100 male and female C57B1/6J mice, an inbred strain with a low incidence of tumours, and C3D2F1/J mice, a hybrid strain with a high incidence of hepatomas in males and a high incidence of mammary tumours in females, were fed endrin (99%) at dietary concentrations of 0.3

Effects on experimental animals and in vitro

or 3 mg/kg from the age of five weeks throughout life. A control group consisted of 200 mice of each sex of each strain. Except for all groups of female animals of the C3D2F1/J strain, this part of the experiment was terminated at the 78th week because of the early occurrence of high numbers of mammary fibroadenomas in 70–90% of control and treated mice. Survival, growth, food intake, and haematology were not impaired. Mice of both strains fed 3 mg/kg diet occasionally developed convulsions in the early stages of feeding but recovered and survived without signs of illness. They generally showed the typical histological changes in the liver characteristic of high doses of chlorinated hydrocarbon insecticides. No effect was observed on mice fed 0.3 mg/kg diet. The tumour incidence and type of tumours were not influenced by the feeding of endrin, and it had no influence on the incidence of fibroadenomas in female C3D2F1/J mice (Witherup et al., 1970).

Groups of 50 B6C3F1 mice of each sex were given endrin in the diet for 80 weeks and were then observed for a further 10 or 11 weeks. The initial doses of endrin (97%) (2.5 and 5 mg/kg of diet) were poorly tolerated by males and were therefore reduced after 25 weeks to 1.2 and 2.5 mg/kg diet for males; but females received 2.5 and 5 mg/kg diet during the whole experiment. The time-weighted average doses were 1.6 and 3.2 mg/kg diet for males and 2.5 and 5.0 mg/kg diet for females. Matched controls consisted of groups of 10 mice of each sex; pooled controls, used for statistical evaluation, consisted of the matched control groups combined with 50 untreated male and 50 untreated female mice from similar bioassays of other chemicals. All surviving mice were killed at 90 or 91 weeks. Mean body weight was not affected, but the survival of males at the high dose was lower than that of the controls. The survival of the low-dose males could not be evaluated due to accidental administration of excessive quantities of endrin to this group during week 66. The tumour (neoplastic lesions in the liver) incidences in the high-dose males were higher than those of the pooled or matched controls, but not significantly so, and the increase was not considered to be related to the administration of endrin (Fredrickson, 1978; NCI, 1978).

8.7.1.2 Rat

A study of groups of 20 male and 20 female Carworth rats administered endrin at 0, 1, 5, 25, 50, and 100 mg/kg of diet was reviewed in Section 8.6.1.1. Bearing in mind the limitations of this study, such as small group sizes and low survival at the high doses, no evidence of an increase in the incidence of neoplasia was found in any of the groups (Treon et al., 1955).

Groups of 50 weanling Osborne-Mendel rats of each sex were fed diets containing endrin (98%) at 2, 6, or 12 mg/kg for 29 months. The control groups consisted of 100 males and 100 females. During the first 10 weeks of the study, only half the nominal dietary concentrations of endrin were fed. Signs of toxicity occurred in a few animals in all treatment groups, mainly in females, and included episodes of tremor and clonic convulsions with 'outcries', the incidence of these signs being dose-related. Weight gain was unaffected, and the survival rates in control and treated rats were similar. The liver:body weight ratios were unaffected. A moderate (not dose-related) increase in the incidence of centrilobular cloudy swelling in the liver and of cloudy swelling of the renal tubular epithelium was observed. The lungs of the animals fed endrin exhibited a moderate increase in the incidence of congestion and focal haemorrhages. The tumour incidence in the treatment groups was comparable with that in control rats, and no difference in the type of tumours was found (Deichmann et al., 1970a,b; Deichmann & MacDonald, 1971).

In a life-time study, groups of 24 male and 24 female Osborne-Mendel rats (22 days old) were fed diets containing endrin at 0, 0.1, 1, 5, 10, or 25 mg/kg. Because 50% of the rats at 25 mg/kg died within the first week, this group was restarted with 32-day-old rats. Survival did not appear to be affected by treatment. The highest incidence of malignant tumours in male and female rats occurred at 0.1 mg/kg, but the malignancies were not dose-related. Treated male rats had a higher incidence of renal disease than controls, but this also was not dose-related (details not available) (Reuber, 1978).

Groups of 50 Osborne-Mendel rats of each sex were fed endrin (97%) in their diet for 80 weeks and then observed for 31 or 34 weeks. Males received doses of 2.5 or 5 mg/kg diet; in females, the initial doses of 5 and 10 mg/kg of diet were poorly tolerated and were reduced after 9 weeks to 2.5 and 5 mg/kg. The time-weighted average doses were 2.5 and 5.0 mg/kg for males and 3 and 6 mg/kg for females. Matched controls consisted of groups of 10 rats of each sex; pooled controls used for statistical evaluation consisted of the matched control groups combined with 40 untreated male and 40 untreated female rats from similar bioassays of other chemicals. All surviving rats were killed at 100–114 weeks. Body weights and survival were not affected by administration of endrin. A slight increase in the

Effects on experimental animals and in vitro

incidences of pituitary and thyroid tumours was observed, but no consistent statistical significance or dose–response relationship was found (Fredrickson, 1978; NCI, 1978).

8.7.1.3 Tumour promotion

No significant increase in the development of preneoplastic changes (hyperplastic nodules) was observed in rat liver after partial hepatectomy and initiation with *N*-nitrosodimethylamine or *N*-2-fluorenylacetamide in combination with the administration of endrin (Ito et al., 1980).

In vitro, endrin at levels of above 2.5 µg/ml appeared to inhibit metabolic cooperation in the hypoxanthineguanine phosphoribosyl transferase system using wild-type 6-thioguanine-sensitive V79 cells and variant 6-thioguanine-resistant cells. Such inhibition is reported to be an index of potential tumour promoting activity, although the test has not been validated (Kurata et al., 1982).

Endrin stimulated protein kinase C activity *in vitro* only slightly, whereas a representative endogenous ligand of protein kinase C, *syn*-1,2-didecanoylglycerol, stimulated protein kinase C to a maximal velocity (Moser & Smart, 1989).

8.7.2 Appraisal of carcinogenicity

One of several studies in mice suggests an increased incidence of nonmalignant tumours in animals of one sex, but this study was considered inadequate for assessing carcinogenicity because an increased number of tumours was seen in controls. A second study using a different mouse strain did not corroborate the increase in tumour incidence. Several long-term feeding studies in rats provide no evidence of a carcinogenic effect of endrin. Its tumour promoting activity was tested *in vitro* using protein kinase C stimulation and ATPase inhibition; the results do not suggest any overwhelming effect in these systems. After a careful review of this evidence, and taking into consideration the fact that most of the data indicate that endrin is not genotoxic, the Task Group concluded that the data are insufficient to indicate that endrin is a carcinogenic hazard to humans.

8.8 Special studies

8.8.1 Nervous system

8.8.1.1 Electrophysiological studies

The effects of endrin on bioelectrogenesis was studied in anaesthetized pigeons and squirrel monkeys with chronically implanted electrodes. Endrin was administered intravenously to pigeons at doses of 0.5–4 mg/kg body weight. Doses of 2–4 mg/kg and higher caused seizure activity throughout the telencephalon; the lower dose levels caused activity only in the ectostriatum, a telecephalic visual projection area. At doses of 0.5–2 mg/kg body weight, endrin caused a specific increase in the evocation of potentials in the ectostriatum by stimulation of the nucleus rotundus, a diencephalic visual projection area. Reticular formation functions were not or little affected. Administration of endrin to squirrel monkeys at doses of 0.2–3 mg/kg body weight on 5 days/week intramuscularly in corn oil and saline emulsion induced characteristic changes in the electroencephalogram (EEG), culminating in electrographic seizures; these were transient and disappeared when endrin administration was stopped. Seizures reappeared under stress conditions, however, several months after endrin treatment (Revzin, 1966, 1980).

Groups of 20–60 Sprague-Dawley rats with previously implanted electrodes were given endrin in peanut oil orally at 0.8, 1.7, or 3.5 mg/kg body weight per day on 5 days/week for 28 weeks. Dose-dependent mortality occurred during the first week and again at the end of the study. Most changes in the EEG were seen after one week of exposure: these included severe bursts of multiple spikes accompanied by clonic convulsions; other animals had runs of spikes without full-fledged convulsions. The convulsions were usually preceded by a period of hyperventilation. After a further week of exposure, the rats showed normal EEG traces. Some irregular slow-wave activity was seen in animals that were moribund in the last month of feeding (Speck & Maaske, 1958).

The convulsive properties of endrin at 1-2 mg/kg body weight were studied by intravenous injection in locally anaesthetized, paralyzed male cats, in which electrodes were placed in the subcortical structures of the brain. Endrin was dissolved in ethanol (which itself stimulates or inhibits the central nervous system, depending on dose). Changes in the EEG and evoked responses were studied. Hypersynchrony, rhythmic bursts of spikes and waves, and isolated spikes characterized the preictal state. Seizures were always bilateral and symmetrical and of a general tonic–clonic type. Responses in sensory and motor cortexes to sensory nerve stimulation were enhanced three to five fold. The authors concluded that endrin is directly toxic to the mammalian nervous system, is a potent rapidly acting convulsant, and does not require metabolic activation to an active metabolite (Joy, 1976).

8.8.1.2 Histopathological studies

Male CD1 Swiss mice were administered endrin or sesame oil daily by intraperitoneal injection in gradually increasing doses of 1.5–4.0 mg/kg for 4–20 days. Electron microscopic examination of sciatic nerve tissue revealed no morphological change in myelinated nerve fibres, myelin, or associated Schwann cells, but morphological alterations were observed in unmyelinated nerve fibres and associated Schwann cells: axons were swollen, microtubules and neurofilaments showed dissolution, axoplasm was replaced by large clear vesicles, vacuolization was present, and Schwann cells and adaxonal spaces also contained vesicles (Walker & Phillips, 1987; abstract only).

8.8.1.3 Neurotransmitter systems

gamma-Aminobutyric acid systems: The role of the inhibitory neurotransmitter of the central nervous system, gamma-aminobutyric acid (GABA), in the production of convulsions is well established. Polychlorocycloalkane insecticides such as endrin have a potent excitatory action on the nervous system, and the interaction between GABA function and endrin has been studied.

Endrin strongly inhibited GABA-dependent ^{36}Cl uptake by mouse brain vesicles, with an IC_{50} (the concentration required to cause 50% inhibition) of 2.8 µmol/litre. Inhibition was confined to that portion of ^{36}Cl uptake that is GABA-dependent. The result demonstrates disruption of GABA ionophore function in mammalian brain, possibly providing the principal mechanism of toxicity (Bloomquist & Soderlund, 1985). In a comparison of the inhibitory potential of several polychlorocycloalkane insecticides on GABA-dependent ^{36}Cl uptake, the most potent inhibitor was 12-ketoendrin, followed by isobenzan, endrin, and then dieldrin, heptachlor epoxide, aldrin, heptachlor and lindane. This order closely parallels their acute toxicities (Bloomquist et al., 1986).

The effect of these chemicals was also studied in the *tert* butylcyclophosphorothioate (TBPS) system, which has been shown to bind convulsants with varying affinities. The IC_{50} for endrin on ^{35}S-TBPS binding was 0.22 µmol/litre and that for 12-ketoendrin, 0.036 µmol/litre. These were the most potent inhibitors of TBPS binding, and there was a significant linear correlation between ^{36}Cl flux and TBPS binding (Bloomquist et al., 1986).

In vitro, endrin inhibited ^{35}S-TBPS binding in tissue from male Swiss-Webster mice with an IC_{50} of 18 nmol/litre (range, 4-90). *In vivo*, doses representing 25, 50, and 100% of the LD_{50} (8 mg/kg intraperitoneally) inhibited ^{35}S-TBPS binding with $IC_{50}s$ of 77 ± 7 nmol/litre (LD_{50}) and 39 ± 6 nmol/litre ($LD_{50}/2$); no inhibition was observed at $LD_{50}/4$, indicating a possible no-observed-adverse-effect level. Brain P2 membranes of treated mice contained endrin and 12-ketoendrin. The finding that the brains of treated mice contained sufficient endrin or its biotransformed products to achieve TBPS binding and that this was correlated with the severity of the poisoning indicates that the acute toxicity of endrin to mammals is regulated by GABA (Cole & Casida, 1986).

GABA-induced ^{36}Cl flux into membrane microsacs was inhibited by endrin at 3.9 ± 0.2 nmol/mg protein, which also suggests that endrin inhibits the function of this receptor (Abalis et al., 1985, 1986). The IC_{50} for ^{36}Cl influx was 0.19 ± 0.06 µM and that for ^{35}S-TBPS binding was 0.003 µM (Gant et al., 1987).

Endrin inhibited both insect and rat GABA receptors in a dose-related, non-competitive manner. It acts in a similar manner on the GABA receptors in the central nervous system of the two species. The blocking action may involve non-competitive binding to an allosteric site associated with the receptor's chloride channel (Wafford et al., 1989a).

Endrin potentially inhibits ^{35}S-TBPS binding to rat brain membranes and also potentiates the protective effect of NaCl (200 mM) against heat inactivation of ^3H-flunitrazepam binding sites on the same membranes. The time courses of heat inactivation of these binding sites in the presence of NaCl and saturating concentrations of endrin revealed monophasic components constituting about 88% of the binding sites (Squires & Saederup, 1989).

Effects on experimental animals and in vitro

Endrin has also been shown to inhibit GABA-ergic function in *Torpedo* fish (Matsumoto et al., 1988), chicken embryos (Seifert, 1988, 1989), the mosquito fish (*Gambusia affinis*) (Bonner & Yarbrough, 1989), and the cockroach (*Periplaneta americana*) (Wafford et al., 1989b).

Other amine systems: Studies on the effects of orally administered endrin on the content of biogenic amines in the brain of rats did not contribute to an understanding of the convulsive action of endrin (Miller & Fink, 1973; Hrdina et al., 1974).

Cyclic AMP metabolism: Endrin did not affect adenylate cyclase activity or inhibit the activity levels of synaptosomal phosphodiesterase, enzymes involved in cyclic AMP metabolism, in rat brain. The authors interpreted their results to support their postulation that organochlorine insecticides exert their neurotoxic action by selective inhibition of ATPases in synaptosomes (Kodavanti et al., 1988).

ATPase systems: Inhibition of rat brain Na^+-K^+ATPase by chlorinated insecticides varied considerably: endrin and dieldrin were the least active in inhibiting both this enzyme and K^+-stimulated *para*-nitrophenyl phosphatase at a concentration of 2×10^{-5} mol/litre. Results of experiments on ATP-$^{32}P_i$ exchange suggest that DDT is a powerful inhibitor of oxidative phosphorylation, which may lead to depletion of ATP. This effect was much less evident with endrin (Folmar, 1978).

Endrin caused about 15% inhibition of the activity of Na^+-K^+ATPase in rat brain synaptosomes at the highest concentration tested, 120 μM, and oligomycin-sensitive Mg^{2+}-ATPase in rat brain synaptosomes was significantly inhibited in a concentration-dependent manner, to a maximal inhibition of 33% at the highest dose. Endrin did not inhibit oligomycin-insensitive Mg^{2+}-ATPase, and it did not affect K^+-stimulated *para*-nitrophenyl phosphatase from rat brain synaptosomes; this enzyme represents the dephosphorylation step of the overall reaction to the Na^+-K^+ATPase. Oligomycin-sensitive Mg^{2+}-ATPase in beef heart mitochondria was significantly inhibited. The results of this study suggest that the ATPase system in rat heart and central nervous system is not selectively inhibited by endrin (Mehrotra et al., 1989).

Sodium channel: It has been demonstrated using voltage clamp techniques in single cells that application of DDT prolongs the sodium current, which in turn decreases the depolarizing after-potential to initiate repetitive after-discharges in the cell. The repetitive after-discharges facilitate synaptic transmission and result in nervous system hyperexcitability, which at the functional level is registered as tremors and eventually convulsions and death (Narahasi, 1987). Even if less than 1% of the sodium channels respond in this manner to insecticides, it is sufficient to cause toxicity in the animal. Narahasi (1987) reported these effects with pyrethroids and a series of DDT analogues; such studies have not been carried out with endrin. Lund & Narahasi (1983) suggested that because of the similarity in the symptomatology of intoxication by the family of organochlorine insecticides, the target site of endrin may also be the sodium channels.

8.8.1.4 Appraisal of effects on the nervous system

The effect of endrin on the nervous system has received attention because it has the well established ability to cause convulsions following acute exposures. Endrin causes considerable changes in EEG activity, which are associated with convulsions, at intramuscular doses in experimental animals as low as 0.2 mg/kg body weight.

The probable underlying mechanisms are associated with a dose-related, non-competitive inhibition of the GABA-ergic neurotransmitter system. This is an inhibitory system, and removal of its action leads to increased excitation in the nervous system. While inhibition of GABA-ergic function is common to a number of polychlorocycloalkane insecticides, endrin, and particularly its metabolite 12-ketoendrin, have been shown to be extremely potent inhibitors of this function. It appears therefore that the acute toxicity of endrin is due to disruption of GABA-related mechanisms.

8.8.2 Cardiovascular system

Studies have been conducted on the physiological effects of endrin on the peripheral vascular system, renal function, renal haemodynamics, and the cardiovascular system of the dog (Emerson et al., 1963, 1964; Reins et al., 1964; Emerson, 1965; Emerson & Hinshaw, 1965; Reins et al., 1966; Hinshaw et al., 1966; Reddy et al., 1967). After a lethal dose of endrin was administered intravenously, most of the effects appeared to be the direct or indirect result of the stimulating action of endrin on the central nervous system. Bradycardia, hypertension, salivation, hyperexcitability, tonic–clonic convulsions, increased body temperature, leukocytosis, haemoconcentration, and decreased blood pH were seen. Elevation of

Effects on experimental animals and in vitro

cerebral venous pressure and cerebrospinal fluid pressure were also prominent features. Increased levels of adrenaline and noradrenaline in blood plasma cause increased venous return and cardiac output and increased arterial blood pressure in the absence of a rise in total peripheral resistance. There was a large increase in total limb vascular resistance and also a decrease in renal blood flow due to arteriolar vasoconstriction. In studies on intact dogs and isolated heart–lung preparations, high doses of endrin appeared to have a toxic action on the left ventricle of the heart, causing sudden left heart failure.

Aldrin, dieldrin, and endrin inhibited rat brain synaptosomal and heart sarcoplasmic reticulum *in vitro* in a concentration-dependent manner. Calmodulin-depleted Ca^{2+} pump activity was insensitive to the action of these compounds. Oral administration of endrin at 0.5–10 mg/kg to rats similarly decreased Ca^{2+} pump activity, in addition to decreasing the levels of calmodulin in both brain and heart, indicating disruption of membrane Ca^{2+} transport mechanisms. Exogenous addition of calmodulin (1–20 μg) effectively reversed the endrin-induced inhibition. Ca^{2+} pump activity in brain is more sensitive to endrin than that in heart. The results indicate that endrin may produce neurotoxic effects by altering calmodulin-regulated calcium-dependent events in neurons (Mehrotra et al., 1989).

8.8.3 Effects on liver enzymes

It is well known that chlorinated hydrocarbon insecticides such as DDT and dieldrin stimulate hepatic microsomal drug metabolism, stimulating the activity of enzymes for the metabolism of drugs and endogenous compounds such as hormones (Kinoshita & Kempf, 1970).

8.8.3.1 Mouse

A single oral, convulsive dose of endrin (20 mg/kg body weight) dissolved in corn oil was administered to 9-week-old male Swiss-Webster mice. Control groups consisted of a group of untreated mice and a group receiving corn oil. When convulsions began, blood serum was examined for serum glutamic oxaloacetic transaminase, serum glutamic pyruvic transaminase, and serum lactic dehydrogenase. The activities of the three enzymes were significantly increased above those seen in the two control groups (Luckens & Phelps, 1969).

After intraperitoneal injection of a single dose of endrin at 6.25 mg/kg body weight to mice, hexobarbital sleeping time was decreased, starting 3 h after the injection and lasting for 3 days (Hart & Fouts, 1963). Stimulating effects on the hepatic mixed-function oxidase system were reported in ICR mice after single oral doses of 4 and 10 mg/kg body weight (Hartgrove et al., 1977).

8.8.3.2 Rat

Feeding Sprague-Dawley rats on diets containing endrin at 1, 5, 25, 50, or 100 mg/kg for 16 weeks caused high mortality in all groups, especially among male rats. The serum alkaline phosphatase concentration was reported to be dose-relatedly increased in all groups as compared to control animals. The effect was clearest in the groups fed 25 mg/kg of diet or more (Nelson et al., 1956).

In strain FW 49 rats, a single oral dose of endrin at 5 mg/kg body weight had no effect on pentobarbital sleeping time; 10 mg/kg caused a significant reduction, which, however, disappeared after 10 days (Schwabe & Wendling, 1967).

Endrin caused a significant shortening of the duration of the paralysis induced by zoxazolamine in male Sprague-Dawley rats aged 5-6 weeks. Endrin was injected intraperitoneally at 2 mg/kg body weight daily for 3 days, and zoxazolamine was injected intraperitoneally on the fourth day (Truhaut et al., 1974).

Male rats given single oral doses of 2.5, 3.75, or 5.0 mg/kg body weight showed no effect on the various parameters (details not given) of mixed-function oxidase activity after 12 h, but the level of microsomal protein and electron transport components per gram of liver were significantly increased after 108 h, in a dose-dependent fashion. Thiopentone and pentobarbital sleeping times were reduced by a 24-h prior intraperitoneal injection of endrin at 5 mg/kg body weight (Kachole & Pawar, 1977).

A single oral dose of endrin at 10 mg/kg body weight to male albino rats increased serum glutamic oxaloacetic transaminase and glutamic pyruvic transaminase activities, and decreased ATPase, acid- and alkaline phosphatase, succinic dehydrogenase, and glucose-6-phosphatase activities significantly 2–48 h after treatment (Meena et al., 1978). After three successive daily oral doses of endrin at 15 mg/kg body weight to Sprague-Dawley rats, significant increases in total lipids and triglycerides in liver and in serum glutamic pyruvic transaminase activity were seen (Borady et al., 1983).

When two groups of six adult female rats were fed 0 or 28.7 µg/kg body weight, endrin accumulated in the liver (5.47 mg/kg), and its concentration in blood increased progressively up to 28 days. Growth was depressed. The activities of the enzymes aspartate amino transferase and alanine amino transferase were slightly increased (Illahi et al., 1986). Similar results were obtained in a study in which rats were fed 20 µg/kg body weight for 28 days (Illahi et al., 1987).

8.8.3.3 Guinea-pig

Groups of six female guinea-pigs were administered three successive intraperitoneal injections of endrin in sunflower oil at 3 mg/kg body weight, and liver and kidneys were studied 24 h after the last injection. Treatment caused a significant increase in liver weight and a decrease in hepatic microsomal protein content; renal weight and renal microsomal protein content were not affected. Hepatic cytochrome b5 and cytochrome-c reductase activities were increased, while cytochrome P450 and total haem levels were significantly decreased. Related to the decrease in cytochrome P450 was a decrease in TPNH-linked aminopyrine-N-demethylation, but an increase in DPNH-linked demethylation was related to the increase in cytochrome b5 and cytochrome-c reductase. Lipid peroxidation was increased in both liver and kidneys (Pawar & Kachole, 1978).

8.8.3.4 In-vitro studies

To test the possibility that phenobarbital induces cytochrome P450p indirectly by increasing the availability of endogenous glucocorticoids in the liver, phenobarbital and phenobarbital-like inducers, including endrin, were added to primary monolayer cultures of adult Sprague-Dawley rat hepatocytes incubated in serum-free medium without glucocorticoids. De-novo synthesis of cytochrome P450p, measured as increased incorporation of ^{3}H-leucine into immunoprecipitable P450p protein, was increased. Endrin at a concentration of 1×10^{-5} M was half as potent as phenobarbital at 2×10^{-3} M (Schuetz et al., 1986).

8.8.4 Miscellaneous studies

Endrin inhibited rabbit muscle lactate dehydrogenase *in vitro* (Hendrickson & Bowden, 1976). Exposure of isolated rat enterocytes to endrin reduced the efficiency of the neuropeptide vasoactive intestinal peptide after stimulation of cyclic AMP accumulation, as was observed with lindane (Carrero et al., 1989).

Endrin at single oral doses of 25 mg/kg body weight or daily doses of 1 mg/kg body weight daily for 8 days induced various shifts in the mobilization of the ions of biologically important metals such as magnesium, iron, zinc, and copper from liver, kidneys, brain, heart, spleen, and blood (Coleman et al., 1968; Lawrence et al., 1968). Rats receiving intraperitoneal injections of 1 mg/kg body weight in peanut oil over periods up to 19 days showed no alteration in the concentrations of serum proteins or serum lipoproteins, separated by paper electrophoresis, or of albumin, alpha 1, alpha 2, beta, or gamma globulins. Protein-bound sialic acid and methylpentose were increased only temporarily; the level of bound hexose increased with time and that of bound hexosamine decreased (Coleman, 1968).

Rats receiving a single oral dose of 50 mg/kg body weight, daily intraperitoneal doses of 2 mg/kg body weight, or daily intramuscular injections of 0.5 or 2.0 mg/kg body weight for 45 days showed increased activity of a number of the enzymes that are involved in gluconeogenesis in liver cells and cells of the renal cortex. A significant decrease was noted in hepatic glycogen, an increase in blood glucose and urea, as well as a significant rise in hepatic and renal pyruvate carboxylase, phosphoenol pyruvate carboxykinase, fructose-1,6-diphosphatase, and glucose-6-phosphatase. Furthermore, endogenous levels of cyclic AMP were increased (Kacew et al., 1973; Singhal & Kacew, 1976).

8.8.5 Factors that influence toxicity

8.8.5.1 Nutrition

The nutritional state of Wistar rats was found to alter their susceptibility to the acute toxic action of endrin. Three groups of approximately 100 rats were fed a normal diet, a diet containing casein as the only source of protein, or a low protein diet for 28 days, and the acute toxicity of endrin was determined after a single intragastric administration. The following

Effects on experimental animals and in vitro

LD_{50} values were calculated: 27 mg, 17 mg, and 7 mg/kg body weight, respectively (Boyd & Stefec, 1969).

8.8.5.2   Potentiation

The acute oral LD_{50}s of equitoxic doses of combinations of 10 pesticides, including endrin, were studied in Swiss mice. No evidence of potentiation was seen with combinations with dieldrin, diazinon, malathion, toxaphene, parathion, DDT, or dioxathion, but more than additive effects, i.e., possible potentiation, were found with chlordane and possibly with aldrin (Keplinger & Deichmann, 1967).

Five groups of 20 male and 20 female Sprague-Dawley rats were fed for 91 days on a diet containing a combination of 15 'persistent' chemicals added at concentrations of 0, 1, 10, 100, and 1000 times the water quality objective applied in Canada. For endrin, these corresponded to 0.002, 0.02, 0.2, and 2.0 µg/kg of diet. No effect on food intake, growth, clinical chemistry, bone marrow, or histopathology were observed. It was concluded that the presence of these chemicals at 1000 times the water quality objective had no toxicological effect (Cote et al., 1985).

Six male and six female Sprague-Dawley rats were fed a control diet or diets containing endrin at 5 or 10 mg/kg, endrin aldehyde at 10 mg/kg, or endrin ketone at 5 mg/kg for 15 days, at which time three to six rats from each treatment group were given a single intraperitoneal dose of carbon tetrachloride at 100 µlitre/kg body weight in corn oil (1 mg/kg). Levels of serum enzymes, bile flow, and biliary excretion of an anionic model compound, phenolphthalein glucuronide, were measured on day 16. Dietary treatment with endrin at either dose level did not elevate serum enzyme levels. Treatment with 5 mg/kg significantly reduced bile flow and a corresponding reduction in phenolphthalein glucuronide excretion, whereas the 10 mg/kg dose reduced only phenolphthalein glucuronide excretion in male rats. Female rats treated with either dose showed a dose-dependent choleretic effect with a commensurate increase in phenolphthalein glucuronide excretion. Treatment of rats with endrin and carbon tetrachloride did not result in potentiation of hepatobiliary functions. The levels of some serum enzymes were elevated (two-fold) in rats given endrin plus carbon tetrachloride over those in rats given endrin or carbon tetrachloride alone, indicating an additive interaction. Dietary treatment with endrin aldehyde slightly increased the levels of serum glutamic oxaloacetic transaminase and glutamic pyruvic transaminase; and endrin ketone induced a small elevation in glutamic pyruvic transaminase levels. Neither compound altered bile flow or biliary phenolphthalein glucuronide excretion. Combination with carbon tetrachloride increased the levels of some serum enzymes (two-fold) over those seen with the aldehyde or the ketone or carbon tetrachloride alone (Young & Mehendale, 1986).

9. EFFECTS ON HUMAN BEINGS

9.1 Exposure of the general population

9.1.1 Acute toxicity

In mild cases of poisoning, dizziness, weakness of the legs, abdominal discomfort, nausea, and vomiting have been reported. Some patients have complained of temporary deafness or were slightly disorientated or aggressive. The onset of poisoning is variable and may occur 0.5–10 h after consumption of contaminated food or contamination of the skin; the interval is usually 1–4 h, depending on the quantity ingested. Severe poisoning is manifested by sudden epileptiform fits, with frothing at the mouth, facial congestion, and violent convulsive movements of the limbs, sometimes leading to dislocation of a shoulder or other injury. The fits may last for several minutes and may be followed by a period of semiconsciousness for 15–30 min or until the next fit. In general, these convulsions occur suddenly, with no prodromal sign or symptom. An uncommon but very serious symptom observed in two children was hyperthermia (41 °C or higher); the high fever was followed by decerebrate rigidity. In fatal cases, death occurs within 2–12 h. In survivors, recovery is rapid, within 24 h, and uneventful, although some patients have complained of headache, dizziness, weakness, and anorexia for several weeks (Davis & Lewis, 1956; Jacobziner & Raybin, 1959; Hoogendam et al., 1962; Hayes, 1963; Weeks, 1967; Hayes, 1982). After clinical recovery, EEG changes consisting of bilateral synchronous theta-wave activity and occasional bilateral synchronous spike and wave complexes, believed to be associated with brain stem irritation, may still be found and may persist for up to several weeks (Hoogendam et al., 1962, 1965; Weeks, 1967).

9.1.2 Poisoning incidents

Hayes (1982) reviewed poisoning cases caused by endrin. Outbreaks of acute intoxication due to endrin have occurred by contamination of flour during transport in railway cars. A first episode, which was well studied, occurred in 1956 in Wales, United Kingdom (Davis & Lewis, 1956): At least 59 people were ill enough to require medical treatment, and at least 100 more had some symptoms, which were not severe enough to require medical advice. No one died. On the basis of the concentration of endrin in bread prepared from the flour (150 mg/kg), Hayes (1963) estimated that

0.20–0.25 mg/kg body weight may cause a single convulsion and that the dose necessary to produce repeated convulsions is about 1 mg/kg body weight. Karplus (1971) estimated the lethal dose in man to be approximately 10 mg/kg body weight.

A few conflicting data are available on the concentration of endrin in the tissues of victims of fatal intoxication. Hayes (1982) quoted levels of 7–10 mg/kg in the liver and 0.7–4.4 mg/kg in the brain; however, 10-fold lower levels were reported in the tissues of autopsied victims of an outbreak of poisoning caused by ingestion of bread prepared from contaminated flour in the Middle East (Curley et al., 1970). In another incident, two sacks of contaminated flour contained endrin at 184.5 and 234.5 mg/kg, and the bread and rolls prepared from the contaminated flour contained 125.67–176.11 mg/kg. The levels of endrin in serum, collected 30 min, 20 h, and 30 h after convulsions in one person were 0.053, 0.038, and 0.021 mg/litre, respectively; three other cases had 0.003–0.004 mg/litre of blood serum 9–19 h after convulsions. One of these three people had no symptoms (Coble et al., 1967). The reported serum or blood levels of endrin associated with convulsions must be interpreted in the context of the rapid removal of endrin from blood and the often significant time lag in taking blood samples after convulsions. When the time between convulsion and blood sampling is long, the endrin levels reported are likely to be much lower than those at the time of the convulsion.

Four outbreaks of endrin intoxication occurred in Doha (Qatar) and Hofuf (Saudi Arabia) in 1967, during which 874 people were hospitalized of whom 26 died; another 500–750 people showed symptoms of intoxication but required no hospitalization. These outbreaks were due to contamination of flour by endrin leaking from drums during shipment. The endrin concentrations found in bread were 48–1807 mg/kg, and those in the blood of patients were 0.007–0.032 mg/litre (Weeks, 1967; Curley et al., 1970).

Between July and September 1984, an epidemic of endrin poisoning occurred in Pakistan, resulting in acute convulsions. In 18 of 21 affected villages surveyed, 70% (106/152) of the cases for which age was known were in children aged 1–9 years; 9.8% (19/194) of the affected people died. A composite sugar sample taken from the houses of three cases contained endrin at 0.04 mg/kg. Endrin was detected in the blood of 12/18 patients, at levels of 0.3–254.0 µg/litre of serum. It was also determined in brain, kidneys, adipose tissue, and liver of one person and found at levels of 1680, 1760, 4010, 1430 µg/kg respectively (Anon., 1984; Hill et al., 1986; Rowley et al., 1987).

Effects on human beings

In mid-March 1988, three members of a family in Orange County, California, USA, became ill within 1 h of eating taquitos (baked corn shell filled with spicy meat and salad). Two of the three had multiple *grand mal* seizures. Subsequently, two other people were reported to have had seizures less than 12 h after eating taquitos. All five patients had obtained the taquitos from the same shop within 5 days. The food was analysed, and the presence of endrin was confirmed but not quantified. The origin of the endrin could not be identified (Anon., 1989).

An episode of acute endrin poisoning was reported in 33 Mexican children, who had sudden seizures without sensory alterations (Singh & West, 1985).

Several other cases have been published of single accidental or intentional intoxications, in children and in adults (Jacobziner & Raybin, 1959; Karplus, 1971). Reddy et al. (1966) described 60 cases of fatal endrin poisoning out of 95 encountered in India after the introduction of endrin in agricultural work as an insecticide in 1959. The majority of the cases were suicidal. Froth, petechial haemorrhages, a kerosene-like smell and massive pulmonary oedema were the characteristic autopsy findings. Respiratory failure was the most common cause of death. The authors concluded that the toxic dose of endrin is 5–50 mg/kg body weight or about 1 g; the lethal dose is about 6 g. In a poisoning case in a 19-year-old male who ingested an unknown amount of endrin, convulsions and gross pulmonary oedema were found (Jedeikin et al., 1979). No histological changes were found in the liver. At least some of the pulmonary changes seen in such cases may be due to aspiration of the petroleum hydrocarbon solvent in formulations of endrin.

A case of polyneuropathy of the Guillain-Barré type was attributed to exposure to a mixture of DDT and endrin. Since convulsions were not recorded, the causal relationship remains doubtful (Jenkins & Toole, 1964).

In a fatal case of endrin poisoning, ingestion of 12 g of endrin by a 49-year-old man caused convulsions (persisting for 4 days), hypersalivation, hyperthermia, renal insufficiency, thrombocytopenia, and recurrent hypotension. Death followed after 11 days due to pulmonary complications (infection and haemorrhage) and hypoxaemia causing bradycardia and cardiac arrest. The endrin concentrations in blood 4 h and 6 and 11 days after ingestion were 450, 86 and 71 µg/litre. Endrin levels in adipose tissue, heart, brain, kidneys, and liver, 11 days after ingestion were 89.5, 0.87, 0.89, 0.55, and 1.32 mg/kg, respectively (Runhaar et al., 1985).

The medical treatment of endrin poisoning is described in Annex II.

9.2 Occupational exposure

9.2.1 Factory workers

No fatal case has been reported due to occupational exposure in manufacturing and formulating plants (Van Raalte, 1965; Jager, 1970), which may be due in part to underreporting but is also certainly due to the fact that occupational exposure involving the absorption of lethal doses occurs rarely under practical circumstances. Furthermore, the rapid metabolism of endrin minimizes build-up of toxic levels in tissues during normal working days.

Several cases of acute, non-fatal poisoning occurred in a manufacturing plant in The Netherlands due to accidental over-exposure to endrin (Jager, 1970). Endrin had been manufactured in this plant since 1957. During the first 9 years of production of aldrin, dieldrin, and endrin in the plant, 17 cases of poisoning with convulsions occurred, five of which involved more than one convulsion. Three of the cases were due to acute over-exposure to endrin among workers who were handling these materials at high concentrations every day. There was no fatality during 1300 man-years of exposure. No evidence was found of skin sensitization, and there was no case of permanent, partial, or complete incapacity. No difference was seen in absenteeism due to illness among these workers in comparison with those in other plants, and the results of liver function tests and complete blood cell counts were within normal limits. In the cases of poisoning, recovery from clinical and neurological signs, including EEG tracings, was rapid and complete (Hoogendam et al., 1962, 1965; Jager, 1970; Versteeg & Jager, 1973).

A series of studies has been published on the results of continuing medical supervision of workers in this plant. A complementary follow-up of 189 workers and of 52 workers who had left employment at the plant for various reasons was published in 1973 (Versteeg & Jager, 1973). These workers had been exposed to endrin for up to 14.5 years in 1973. In agreement with data published from a study of 71 workers in an endrin manufacturing plant in the USA (Hayes & Curley, 1968), endrin was not found in the blood of these workers, except in cases of accidental, acute over-exposure. Medical supervision of workers employed in the manufacture and formulation of endrin and other pesticides for 1–19 years (average, 12 years), data on absenteeism, the results of tests for liver function and blood chemistry, blood morphology, urine analysis, the occurrence of sensitization, the pattern and course of EEG changes in cases of poisoning, other medical studies (including electrocardiography, chest x rays, blood pressure, body weight), and the incidence and pattern of diseases, including the occurrence of malignant growths, showed no difference between workers exposed to endrin and other chemical plant operators. Residues of endrin were not found in plasma (< 3 μg/litre) or in adipose tissue (< 0.03 mg/kg).

A significant difference was found between workers exposed to aldrin and dieldrin only, workers not exposed to insecticides, and workers exposed to endrin only: endrin workers had lower blood levels of the DDT metabolite *para,para'*-DDE than the other workers, and the levels were lower than those in the general population of the surrounding area, although DDT and related compounds had never been manufactured in the plant. A second parameter that was compared was excretion of 6-beta-hydrocortisol in the urine. (Increased activity of the drug-metabolizing enzyme system increases the activity of the oxidative pathway by which 6-beta-hydroxylase converts endogenous cortisol to 6-beta-hydrocortisol and thus, relatively, diminishes the contribution of the reductive pathway, leading to excretion of 17-hydroxycorticosteroids.) The ratio of the urinary excretion of 6-beta-hydroxycortisol to that of 17-hydroxysteroids was significantly higher in the endrin workers than in workers not exposed to endrin (Jager, 1970).

A third parameter of this enzyme system that was studied was urinary excretion of D-glucaric acid (an end-product of the glucuronic acid pathway in the liver), which has been shown to increase after exposure to microsomal enzyme-stimulating compounds, like endrin (Hunter et al., 1971; Notten & Henderson, 1975). In the endrin workers, urinary excretion of D-glucaric acid after a week of exposure increased significantly over pre-exposure levels and those in a control group of workers. Excretion diminished again after 3 days without exposure (Hunter et al., 1972; Ottevanger & Van Sittert, 1979; Vrij-Standhardt et al., 1979; Van Sittert, 1985).

Since *anti*-12-hydroxyendrin is the only metabolite found in the urine of endrin-exposed workers, a study was initiated to find whether there is a correlation between the quantity of this metabolite and that of D-glucaric acid excreted in the urine. A positive relationship was found between excretion of the endrin metabolite and of D-glucaric acid after 7 days. After exposure was discontinued, excretion of *anti*-12-hydroxyendrin decreased faster than that of D-glucaric acid. The fact that endrin-exposed workers had D-glucaric acid levels within the normal range after 6 weeks indicates that enzyme induction in endrin workers is reversible. The authors concluded that a urinary level of *anti*-12-hydroxyendrin of 0.130 µg/g of creatinine is the threshold exposure level, below which enzyme induction is not produced (Ottevanger & Van Sittert, 1979; Van Sittert, 1985). Endrin did not increase total urinary porphyrin excretion over that in a control group of employees (Strik, 1979; Nagelsmit et al., 1979; Vrij-Standhardt et al., 1979).

In a follow-up mortality study of the same group of workers, vital status and cause of death were assessed for 232 of a group of more than 1000 workers. This group was selected because they had experienced high exposures in the initial years of manufacture and formulation and because of the long periods of exposure (mean, 11 years; range, 4–27) and observation (mean, 24 years; range, 4–29). Total observed mortality was 25, whereas 38 deaths were expected on the basis of mortality statistics for the male Dutch population. Of the nine cancer deaths, three were due to lung cancer; the remaining six were due to cancers of stomach, pancreas, bladder, and kidney, multiple myeloma, and cerebral glioma. It was concluded that the pesticides manufactured had no specific carcinogenic activity (Ribbens, 1985).

9.2.2 Dose–response relationships

It has not been possible to establish a dose–response relationship between single or repeated oral exposures and endrin concentrations in blood, adipose tissue, or organs and severity of intoxication, because the actual oral intake in the accidental cases was not known, and the onset of symptoms of intoxication and the time of measuring concentrations of endrin in blood, organs, or tissues were not comparable (Davis & Lewis, 1956; Hayes, 1963; Coble et al., 1967; Weeks, 1967; Curley et al., 1970; Karplus, 1971; Hayes, 1982; Anon., 1984).

Effects on human beings

Blood samples have been analysed in three cases of acute overexposure (Table 28): A formulator and an operator were accidentally splashed with a 20% endrin emulsifiable concentrate, which was washed off within 10 min. Neither developed signs or symptoms of intoxication. The third case was in a formulator who handled technical-grade endrin powder without wearing a dust-mask. He had convulsions 4 h after starting work, but after treatment recovered fully the next day. Blood samples from four colleagues working next to him, but wearing dust-masks, were also examined. The author estimated that the threshold level of endrin in the blood below which no sign or symptom of intoxication occurs is 50–100 µg/litre and that the half-life of endrin in blood is in the order of 24 h (Jager, 1970).

9.2.3 *Exposures to mixtures*

A retrospective mortality study was carried out on workers employed in the manufacture of heptachlor and endrin in a plant in Tennessee, USA, between 1952 and 1976. The study comprised 835 men who had worked for more than 3 months up to 20 years at the plant. No overall excess of deaths from cancer was found; however, there was an excess of deaths from cerebrovascular disease (7 observed, 2.3 expected) (Wang & MacMahon, 1979).

A further retrospective cohort study was conducted to examine the mortality of workers employed in the manufacture of chlordane, heptachlor, DDT, aldrin/dieldrin, and endrin in a plant in Colorado, USA, where endrin was manufactured from 1953 until 1965. Approximately 2100 workers who had been employed for at least 6 months in the plants were involved. No excess of cerebrovascular disease was observed (Ditraglia et al., 1981).

Neither study proves conclusively that exposure to these organochlorine insecticides is associated with increased prevalence of malignancy or other cause of death, but they are limited in design and in the desciption of exposure.

A field study was carried out in 1983 in the Ivory Coast to assess the health hazards associated with the handling and application by hand-held sprayers of an ultra-low volume formulation consisting of endrin at 85 g/litre, DDT at 333 g/litre, and methylparathion at 85 g/litre in petroleum solvent. Groups of five or six farmers sprayed 3 litre/ha of the formulation

Table 28. Concentrations of endrin in blood from acutely over-exposed workers

Case	Time of first sampling	Endrin concentration (µg/litre)				
		First sample	12 h later	24 h later	36 h later	5 days later
Formulator	1 h after accident	90				ND
Operator	40 min after accident	27	25		ND	
Formulator without dust-mask	Directly after convulsion	80		20		ND
Four colleagues with dust-masks	Same time time as above	ND-10				

ND, not detectable (< 5 µg/litre)

4–6 weeks after sowing cotton and again 15 or 30 days after the first application. The spray apparatus was filled and cleaned by the same men. The recommended protective clothing was worn only rarely, and the handling and application techniques were careless, resulting in many cases in appreciable skin contamination. No adverse health effect was observed. Absorption of endrin was monitored by measuring the concentration of *anti*-12-hydroxyendrin in spot samples of urine collected about 20 h after spraying. The mean concentrations after the first, second, and third applications were 0.34 (range, 0.04–0.59), 0.52 (range, 0.09–1.4), and 0.45 mg/g of creatinine (range, 0.0–0.92). One person who had handled and sprayed the formulation carefully still had *anti*-12-hydroxyendrin in the urine after the third application, but at a very low level (0.03 mg/g of creatinine). Measurements of *para*-nitrophenol, a metabolite of methylparathion, in urine indicated that the rate of metabolism of methylparathion was increased as a result of enzyme induction by endrin in the liver (Kummer & Van Sittert, 1984, 1986). It was concluded that endrin accumulated in most of the farmers after three applications within a short period. An increase to toxic levels might result if spraying were more frequent and at shorter intervals and if the recommended clothing was not worn.

Effects on human beings

9.2.4 Appraisal of effects of occupational exposures

Endrin is a very toxic compound. Several episodes of fatal and non-fatal poisoning have occurred, mostly from accidental contamination of food and also from intentional (suicidal) ingestion. The lethal oral dose is estimated to be 10 mg/kg body weight. In non-fatal cases, recovery is rapid and complete within a few days. The oral dose that causes a single convulsion is estimated to be 0.25 mg/kg body weight, and that which induces repeated convulsions, 1.0 mg/kg body weight.

Exposure of workers to endrin for long periods did not induce adverse effects that were attributed to this compound, although occasional cases of acute, non-fatal intoxication due to accidental over-exposure have occurred. Endrin was not detected in the blood of workers exposed to endrin at < 3.0 µg/litre. The threshold level of endrin in blood that results in intoxication is estimated to be 50–100 µg/litre. Absorption of a toxic dose is therefore unlikely during occupational exposure if recommended controls and precautions are used. In fatal cases, endrin concentrations in blood as high as 450 µg/litre have been reported; however, it is not possible to establish a dose–response relationship. Since endrin is not normally found in air, water, or food, except under conditions of contamination, exposure of the general population is not significant.

10. PREVIOUS EVALUATIONS BY INTERNATIONAL BODIES

Endrin was evaluated by the Joint FAO/WHO Expert Committee on Pesticide Residues in 1963, 1965, and 1970 (FAO/WHO, 1964, 1965, 1971). In 1970, the Committee established an acceptable daily intake (ADI) for humans of 0–0.0002 mg/kg body weight, which was based on the level that causes no toxicological effect in rats and dogs, 1 mg/kg of diet (equivalent to 0.05 mg/kg body weight per day in rats and 0.025 mg/kg body weight per day in dogs).

The Joint FAO/WHO Codex Alimentarius Commission has published maximum residue limits for endrin (Table 29; (FAO/WHO, 1986b).

Table 29. Codex maximum limits for the sum of residues of endrin and delta-ketoendrin

Commodity	Maximum residue limit (mg/kg product)
Apples	0.02[a]
Barley	0.02[a]
Cottonseed	0.1
Cottonseed oil (crude)	0.1
Cottonseed oil (edible)	0.02[a]
Eggs (without shells)	0.2
Meat (carcass fat)	0.1[b]
Milk	0.0008[b]
Poultry (carcass fat)	1
Rice (husked or polished)	0.02[a]
Sorghum	0.02[a]
Sweet maize	0.02[a]
Wheat	0.02[a]

[a] At or near the limit of detection
[b] Extraneous residue limit

The International Agency for Research on Cancer (IARC) concluded in 1974 and 1987 that there was inadequate evidence for the carcinogenicity of endrin in experimental animals and that the evidence from studies in humans was inadequate. Endrin was therefore classified in Group 3: not classifiable as to its carcinogenicity to humans (IARC, 1974, 1987).

Previous evaluations by international bodies

In 1988, the Pesticide Development and Safe Use Unit, Division of Vector Biology and Control, WHO, classified technical-grade endrin as highly hazardous in normal use (WHO, 1992). A data sheet on endrin was issued in 1978 (WHO/FAO, 1975).

REFERENCES

Abalis IM, Eldefrawi ME, & Eldefrawi AT (1985) High-affinity stereospecific binding of cyclodiene insecticides and γ-hexachlorocyclohexane to γ-aminobutyric acid receptors of rat brain. Pestic Biochem Physiol, **24**: 95–102.

Abalis IM, Eldefrawi ME, & Eldefrawi AT (1986) Effects of insecticides on GABA-induced chloride influx into rat brain microsacs. J Toxicol Environ Health, **18**: 13–23.

Abbott DC, Harrison RB, Tatton JO'G, & Thomson J (1966) Organochlorine pesticides in the atmosphere. Nature, **211**(5046): 259–261.

Abbott DC, Goulding R, & Tatton JO'G (1968) Organochlorine pesticide residues in human fat in Great Britain. Br Med J, **iii**: 146–149.

Abbott DC, Holmes DC, & Tatton JO'G (1969) Pesticide residues in the total diet in England and Wales, 1966–67. Organochlorine pesticide residues in the total diet. J Sci Food Agric, **20**(4): 245–259.

Abbott DC, Collins GB, & Goulding R (1972) Organochlorine pesticide residues in human fat in United Kingdom. Br Med J, ii: 553–556

Abdel-Razik M, Marzouk MAH, Mowafy LE, & Abdel-Kader MA (1988) Pesticide residues in the River Nile water, Egypt. Pak J Sci Ind Res, **31**(11): 795–797.

Abdou SM, Abdel-Gawaad AA, Abdel-Amaim E, Abdel-Hady SM, & El-Alfy MB (1983) Organochlorine pesticide residues in buffaloes milk in Kalubia province and the effect of the presence of insecticides on coagulation time. Egypt J Dairy Sci, **11**: 197-203.

Acker L & Schulte E (1974) [Chlorinated hydrocarbons in human fat.] Naturwissenschaften, **61**: 32 (in German).

Albanis TA, Pomonis PJ, & Sdoukos AT (1986) Seasonal fluctuations of organochlorine and triazines pesticides in the aquatic system of Ioannina Basin (Greece). Sci Total Environ, **58**: 243-253.

Albers PH, Sileo L, & Mulhern BM (1986) Effects of environmental contaminants on snapping turtles of a tidal wetland. Arch Environ Contam Toxicol, **15**: 39–49.

Albert LA (1990) Environmental contamination in Mexican food. In: Hriagu JO & Simmons MS ed., Food contamination from environmental sources. New York, John Wiley and Sons, pp 542–577.

References

Albert L, Mendez F, Cebrian ME, & Portales A (1980) Organochlorine pesticide residues in human adipose tissue in Mexico. Results of a preliminary study in three Mexican cities. Arch Environ Health, **35**(5): 262-269.

Albert LA, Vega P, & Nava E (1982) [Organochlorine pesticides. VI. Organochlorine pesticide residues in Mexican evaporated milks.] Biotica, **7**(3): 473-482 (in Spanish).

Alford-Stevens AL, Eichelberger JW, & Budde WL (1988) Multi-laboratory study of automated determination of polychlorinated biphenyls and chlorinated pesticides in water, soil and sediment by gas chromatography/mass spectrometry. Environ Sci Technol, **22**: 304-312.

Ali SL (1986) [Pesticide residues and traces of heavy metals in cod liver oil.] Pharm Ztg, **131**(38): 2288-2290 (in German).

Al-Omar MA, Al-Ogaily NH, Tawfiq SJ, & Al-Bassoumy M (1985a) Residue levels of organochlorine insecticides in sewage plant effluent. J Biol Sci Res, **16**(1): 145-151.

Al-Omar MA, Tameesh AH, & Al-Ogaily NH (1985b) Dairy product contamination with organochlorine insecticide residues in Bagdad district. J Biol Sci Res, **16**(1): 133-144.

Altmeier G & Korte F (1969) [Contributions to ecological chemistry (XXIV). Metabolism of endrin-^{14}C in perfused rats' livers.] Tetrahedron Lett, **49**: 4269-4271 (in German).

Anderson A (1986) Monitoring and biased sampling of pesticide residues in fruits and vegetables. Methods and results, 1981-1984. Var Foda, **38**(Suppl. 1): 8-55.

Anderson RL & Defoe DL (1980) Toxicity and bioaccumulation of endrin and methoxychlor in aquatic invertebrates and fish. Environ Pollut (Ser A), **22**: 111-121.

Anderson HH, Hine CH, Kodama JJ, & Critchlow JK (1953) Class B Determination on HI-1185 Endrin Emulsifiable Concentrate, San Francisco, University of California, School of Medicine (UC Report No. 213).

Ang C, Meleady K, & Wallace L (1989) Pesticide residues in drinking water in the north coast region of New South Wales, Australia, 1986-87. Bull Environ Contam Toxicol, **42**: 595-602.

Anon. (1964) Report on investigation of fish kills in Lower Mississippi River, Atchafalaya River and Gulf of Mexico. Washington, DC, US Department of Health, Education, and Welfare, Public Health Service, Division of Water Supply and Pollution Control.

Anon (1979) Determination of residues of organochlorine pesticides in animal fats and eggs. Report of the committee for analytical methods for residues of pesticides and veterinary products in foodstuffs of the Ministry of Agriculture, Fisheries and Food. Analyst, **104**: 425-433.

Anon. (1984) Acute convulsions associated with endrin poisoning—Pakistan. Morb Mortal Wkly Rep, **33**(49): 687–695.

Anon. (1988a) Introduction—US Environmental Protection Agency Office of Drinking Water health advisories. Rev Environ Contam Toxicol, **104**: 1–8.

Anon. (1988b) Endrin. Rev Environ Contam Toxico,l **104**: 103–114.

Anon. (1989) Endrin poisoning associated with taquito ingestion, California. Morb Mortal Wkly Rep, **38**(19): 345–347.

Argyle RJ, Williams GC, & Dupree HK (1973) Endrin uptake and release by fingerling channel catfish (*Ictalurus punctatus*). J Fish Res Board Canada, **30**(11): 1743–1744.

Arthur RD, Cain JD, & Barrentine BF (1976) Atmospheric levels of pesticides in the Mississippi Delta. Bull Environ Contam Toxicol, **15**(2): 129–134.

Atkins EL, Greywood EA, & MacDonald RL (1973) Toxicity of pesticides and other agricultural chemicals to honey bees: Laboratory studies. Riverside, University of California, Department of Entomology (Rev. 9/73 (M-16)).

Atuma SS (1985) Accumulation of organochlorine insecticides in the blood of the general population of Nigeria. Toxicol Environ Chem,**10**: 77–82.

Baldwin MK & Hutson DH (1980) Analysis of human urine for a metabolite of endrin by chemical oxidation and gas-liquid chromatography as an indicator of exposure to endrin. Analyst, **105**: 60–65.

Baldwin MK, Robinson J, & Parke DV (1970) Metabolism of endrin in the rat. J Agric Food Chem, **18**(6): 1117–1123.

Baldwin MK, Davis RA, & Burns DT (1973) Structural studies and photochemical rearrangement of an animal metabolite of HEOD, the active component of dieldrin. Pestic Sci, **4**: 227–237.

Baldwin MK, Crayford JV, Hutson DH, & Street DL (1976) The metabolism and residues of ^{14}C-endrin in lactating cows and laying hens. Pestic Sci, **7**(6): 575–594.

Barcelo D & Puignou LG (1987) [Pesticide residue in Spanish U.H.T. milks determined by high resolution gas chromatography.] Rev Agroquim Tecnol Aliment, **27**(4): 583–589 (in Spanish).

Barnett RW, D'Ercole AJ, Cain JD, & Arthur RD (1979) Organochlorine pesticide residues in human milk samples from women living in northwest and northeast Mississippi, 1973-75. Pestic Monit J, **13**(2): 47–51.

Barth RAJ (1967) Pesticide toxicity in primates. Tulane, University of Louisiana, Division of Hygiene and Tropical Medicine (Thesis).

References

Barthel WF, Hawthorne JC, Ford JH, Bolton GC, McDowell LL, Grissinger EH, & Parsons DA (1969) Pesticide residues in sediments of the Lower Mississippi River and its tributaries. Pestic Monit J, 3(1): 8–68.

Batterton JC, Boush JC, & Matsumura F (1971) Growth response of blue-green algae to aldrin, dieldrin, endrin and their metabolites. Bull Environ Contam Toxicol, 6(6): 589–594.

Becker DM & Sieg CH (1987) Egg shell quality and organochlorine residues in eggs of merlins *Falco columbarius* in southeastern Montana. Can Field-Nat, 101: 369–372.

Bedford CT (1974) Von Baeyer/IUPAC names and abbreviated chemical names of metabolites and artifacts of aldrin (HHDN), dieldrin (HEOD) and endrin. Pestic Sci, 5: 473–489.

Bedford CT & Harrod RK (1973) Synthesis of *anti*-12-hydroxyendrin and 12-ketoendrin, the two major mammalian metabolites of endrin. Chemosphere, 4: 163–168.

Bedford CT & Hutson DH (1976) The comparative metabolism in rodents of the isomeric insecticides dieldrin and endrin. Chem Ind, 1976: 440–447.

Bedford CT, Harrod RK, Hoadley EC, & Hutson DH (1975a) The metabolic fate of endrin in the rabbit. Xenobiotica, 5(8): 485–500.

Bedford CT, Hutson DH, & Natoff IL (1975b) The acute toxicity of endrin and its metabolites to rats. Toxicol Appl Pharmacol, 33: 115–121.

Bedford CT, Crane AE, & Harrod RK (1986a) Synthesis and confirmation of structure of four mammalian metabolites of dieldrin and endrin. Pestic Sci, 17: 659–667.

Bedford CT, Crane AE, Smith EH, & Wellard NK (1986b) Synthesis of endrin metabolites. Part. 2: Total synthesis and confirmation of the structure of 3-hydroxyendrin. Pestic Sci, 17: 33–47.

Belisle AA, Reichel WL, Locke LN, Lamont TG, Mulhern BM, Prouty RM, DeWolf RB, & Cromartie E (1972) Residues in fish, wildlife and estuaries. Pestic Monit J, 6: 133–138.

Benes V & Sram R (1969) Mutagenic activity of some pesticides in *Drosophila melanogaster*. Ind Med, 38(12): 442–444.

Bennett RO & Wolke RE (1987a) The effect of sublethal endrin exposure on rainbow trout, *Salmo gairdneri* Richardson. I. Evaluation of serum cortisol concentrations and immune responsiveness. J Fish Biol, 31(3): 375–385.

Bennett RO & Wolke RE (1987b) The effect of sub-lethal endrin exposure on rainbow trout, *Salmo gairdneri* Richardson. II. The effect of altering serum cortisol concentrations on the immune response. J Fish Biol, 31(3): 387–394.

Benson WR (1969) Note on nomenclature of dieldrin and related compounds. J Assoc Off Anal Chem, **52**(5): 1109–1111.

Beyerbach M, Buthe A, Heidmann WA, Dettmer R, & Knuwer H (1987) [Chlorinated hydrocarbons in eggs and livers of rooks (*Corvus frugilegus*) from rookeries in Lower Saxony (northern Germany).] J Ornitol, **128**(3): 277–290 (in German with English summary).

Beyerbach M, Buthe A, Heidmann WA, Knuwer H, & Russel-Sinn HA (1988) [The burden of dieldrin and other chlorinated hydrocarbons on the lapwing (*Vanellus vanellus*).] J Ornitol, **129**(3): 353–361 (in German).

Bhowmik G (1978) Pretreating properties of endrin on plant chromosomes. Letter to the Editor. Curr Sci, **47**(15): 546–547.

Bianchi A, Tateo F, Nava C, Tateo S, Santamaria L, Berte F, & Santagati G (1988) Presence of organophosphate and organochlorine pesticides in the milk of women. Med Biol Environ, **16**: 931–942.

Biberhofer J & Stevens RJJ (1987) Organochlorine contaminants in ambient waters of Lake Ontario. Ottawa, Inland Water Directorate, Waters Quality Branch, pp. 1–11 (Can Sci Ser (87) V51.159).

Biehl ML & Buck WB (1987) Chemical contaminants: their metabolism and their residues. J Food Prot, **50**(12): 1058–1073.

Bloomquist JR & Soderlund DM (1985) Neurotoxic insecticides inhibit GABA-dependent chloride uptake by mouse brain vesicles. Biochem Biophys Res Commun, **133**(1): 37–43.

Bloomquist JR, Adams PM, & Soderlund DM (1986) Inhibition of gamma-aminobutyric acid-stimulated chlorine flux in mouse brain vesicles by polychlorocycloalkane and pyrethroid insecticides. Neurotoxicology, **7**(3): 11–20.

Blus LJ (1978) Short-tailed shrews: toxicity and residue relationship of DDT, dieldrin and endrin. Arch Environ Contam Toxicol, **7**: 83–98.

Blus LJ, Joanen T, Belisle AA, & Prouty RM (1975) The brown pelican and certain environmental pollutants in Louisiana. Bull Environ Contam Toxicol, **13**: 646–655.

Blus L, Cromartie E, McNease L, & Joanen T (1979) Brown pelican: population status, reproductive success, and organochlorine residues in Louisiana, 1971-1976. Bull. Environ Contam Toxicol, **22**: 128–135.

Blus LJ, Henny CJ, Kaiser TE, & Grove RA (1983) Effects on wildlife from use of endrin in Washington State orchards. In: Fox GA & Hall RJ ed. Transactions of the 48th North American Wildlife Conference on Environmental Contaminants and Wildlife. Washington, DC, Wildlife Management Institute, pp. 159–174.

References

Blus LJ, Henny CJ, & Grove RA (1989) Rise and fall of endrin usage in Washington State fruit orchards: effects on wildlife. Environ Pollut, **60**: 331–349.

Boellstorff DE, Ohlendorf HM, Anderson DW, O'Neill EJ, Keith JO, & Prouty RM (1985) Organochlorine chemical residues in white pelicans and western grebes from the Klamath Basin, California. Arch. Environ Contam Toxicol, **14**: 485–493.

Bollag JM & Henninger NM (1976) Influence of pesticides on denitrification in soil and with an isolated bacterium. J Environ Qual, **5**(1): 15–18.

Bollen WB & Tu CM (1971) Influence of endrin on soil microbial populations and their activity. Washington, DC, US Department of Agriculture, Forest Service, pp 1–4 (Research Paper PNW 114).

Bonner JC & Yarbrough JD (1989) Role of the brain t-butyl-bicyclophosphorothionate receptor in vertebrate resistance to endrin, 1,1,1-trichloro-2,2-bis(p-chlorophenyl)ethane and cypermethrin. J Pharmacol Exp Ther, **249**(1): 149–154.

Borady AMA, Mikhail TH, Awadailah R, Ibrahim KA, & Kamar GAR (1983) Effect of some insecticides on fat metabolism and blood enzymes in rats. Egypt J Anim Prod, **23**(1–2): 33–44.

Boyd EM & Stefec J (1969) Dietary protein and pesticide toxicity with particular reference to endrin. Can Med Assoc J, **101**: 335–339.

Braun F (1985) [PCN and chlorine-based pesticides in some Bavarian rivers.]. Munch. Beitr. Abwasser Fisch Flussbiol, **39**: 115–124 (in German).

Breidenbach AW, Gunnerson CG, Kawahara FK, Lichtenberg JJ, & Green RS (1967) Chlorinated hydrocarbon pesticides in major river basins, 1957–65. Public Health Rep, **82**(2): 139–156.

Brodtmann NV. Jr (1976) Continuous analysis of chlorinated hydrocarbon pesticides in the Lower Mississippi River. Bull Environ Contam Toxicol, **15**(1): 33–39.

Brooks GT (1969) The metabolism of diene-organochlorine (cyclodiene) insecticides. Residue Rev, **27**: 81–138.

Brooks GT (1974) Chlorinated insecticides, technology and application. Cleveland, Ohio, CRC Press, vol. 1, pp 85–99 & vol 2, pp 94–97.

Brooks TM (1976) Mutagenicity studies with endrin in the host-mediated assay. Unpublished report No. TLGR.0112.76, Sittingbourne, Kent, Shell Research, submitted to WHO by Shell.

Bunck CM, Prouty RM, & Krynitsky AJ (1987) Residues of organochlorine pesticides and polychlorobiphenyls in starlings (*Sturnus vulgaris*), from the continental United States, 1982. Environ Monit Assess, **8**: 59–75.

Burton WB & Pollard GE (1974) Rate of photochemical isomerization of endrin in sunlight. Bull Environ Contam Toxicol, **12**(1): 113–116.

Butler PA (1963) Commercial fisheries investigations. Washington DC, US Department of the Interior, Fish and Wildlife Service, pp 11–25 (Circular No. 167).

Butler PA (1973) Organochlorine residues in estuarine mollusks, 1965–1972. Pestic Monit J, **6**(4): 238–362.

Cabral JRP, Raitano F, Mollner T, Bronczyk S, & Shubik P (1979) Acute toxicity of pesticides in hamsters. Abstract: Eighteenth Annual Meeting No. 384. Toxicol Appl Pharmacol, **48**: A192.

Caceres O, Tundisi JG, & Castellan OAM (1987) Residues of organochloric pesticides in reservoirs in Sao Paulo State. Cienc Cult, **39**(3): 259–264.

Camanzo J, Rice CP, Jude DJ, & Rossmann R (1987) Organic priority pollutants in near-shore fish from 14 Lake Michigan tributaries and embayments, 1983. J Great Lakes Res, **13**(3): 296–309.

Cantoni C, Fabbris F, Rogledi R, & Campagnari A (1988) [Organochlorine pesticides in foods of animal origin found during the 1985–1987 biennium.] Ind Aliment, **27**(1): 6–8 (in Italian).

Carey AE & Kutz FW (1985) Trends in ambient concentrations of agrochemicals in humans and the environment of the United States. Environ Monit Assess, **5**(2): 155–163.

Carey AE, Gowen JA, Tai H, Mitchell WG, & Wiersma GB (1978) Pesticide residue levels in soils and crops, 1971—national soils monitoring program (III). Pestic Monit J, **12**(3): 117–136.

Carline RF & Lawal MV (1985) Contaminants and bilateral asymmetry in yellow perch. Environ Toxicol Chem, **4**: 543–547.

Carrero I, Fernandez-Moreno MD, Perez-Albarsanz MA, & Prieto JC (1989) Lindane effect upon the vasoactive intestinal peptide receptor/effector system in rat enterocytes. Biochem Biophys Res Commun, **159**(3): 1391–1396.

Carter BI & Simpson BJE (1978) Toxicity of insecticides: The acute oral and percutaneous toxicities of two endrin bleed samples and of technical endrin in Shellsol A and in toluene. Unpublished report No. TLTR.0001.78, Sittingbourne, Kent, Shell Research, submitted to WHO by Shell.

References

Casper VL (1967) Galveston Bay pesticide study—water and oyster samples analyzed for pesticide residues following mosquito control program. Pestic Monit J, 1(3): 13–15.

Casteel SW & Cook WO (1985) Endrin toxicosis in a cat. J Am Vet Med Assoc, 186(9): 988–989.

Castonguay M, Dutil J-D, & Desjardins C (1989) Distinction between American eels (*Anguilla rostrata*) of different geographical origins on the basis of their organochlorine contaminant levels. Can J Fish Aquat Sci, 46: 836–843.

Celeste M de F & Caceres O (1987) [Chlorinated pesticide residues in waters of Ribeirão do Lobo (Broa) reservoir and its tributaries.] Cienc Cult, 39(1): 66–70 (in Portuguese with English summary).

Cetinkaya M (1988) [Organochloro-pesticide residues in tobacco from European cigarette brands.] Chem Mikrobiol Technol Lebensm, 11: 100–103 (in German with English summary).

Cetinkaya M & Schenek A (1987) [Investigation of organochloro-pesticide residues in various raw cotton samples.] Chem Mikrobiol Technol, Lebensm, 10: 150–153 (in German with English summary).

Chau ASY (1974) Confirmation of pesticide residues identity. VII. Solid matrix derivation procedure for the simultaneous confirmation of heptachlor and endrin residues in the presence of large quantities of polychlorinated biphenyls. J Assoc Off Anal Chem, 57(3): 585–591.

Chau ASY & Cochrane WP (1969) Cyclodiene chemistry. III. Derivative formation for the identification of heptachlor, heptachlorepoxide, cis-chlordane, trans-chlordane, dieldrin and endrin pesticide residues by gaschromatography. J Assoc Off Anal Chem, 52: 1220–1226.

Chau ASY & Cochrane WP (1971) Chromous chloride reductions. VI. Derivative formation for the simultaneous identification of heptachlor and endrin pesticide residues by gas chromatography. J Assoc Off Anal Chem, 54(5): 1124–1131.

Chernoff N, Kavlock RJ, Hanisch RC, Whitehouse DA, Gray JA, Gray LE Jr, & Sovocool GW (1979) Perinatal toxicity of endrin in rodents. I. Fetotoxic effects of prenatal exposure in hamsters. Toxicology, 13: 155–165.

Clark DR Jr & Krynitsky A (1978) Organochlorine residues and reproduction in the little brown bat, Laurel, Maryland—June 1976. Pestic. Monit J, 12(3): 113–116.

Clark DR Jr, Laval RK, & Krynitsky AJ (1980) Dieldrin and heptachlor residues in dead gray bats, Franklin County, Missouri—1976 versus 1977. Pestic Monit J, 13(4): 137–140.

Clawson RL & Clark DR (1989) Pesticide contamination of endangered gray bats and their food base in Boone County, Missouri, 1982. Bull Environ Contam Toxicol, **42**: 431–437.

Coble Y, Hildebrandt P, Davis J, Raasch F, & Curley A (1967) Acute endrin poisoning. J Am Med Assoc, **202**: 489–493.

Cole LM & Casida JE (1986) Polychlorocycloalkane insecticide-induced convulsions in mice in relation to disruption of the GABA-regulated chloride ionophore. Life Sci, **39**: 1855–1862.

Cole JF, Klevay LM, & Zavon MR (1970) Endrin and dieldrin: a comparison of hepatic excretion in the rat. Toxicol Appl Pharmacol, **16**: 547–555.

Coleman RL (1968) Endrin induced alterations in bound carbohydrates in rat serum. Bull Environ Contam Toxicol, **3**(6): 348–353.

Coleman RL, Lawrence CH, & Sowell WL (1968) Trace metal alterations following subacute exposure to endrin. Bull. Environ Contam Toxicol, **3**(5): 284–295.

Cook WO & Casteel SW (1985) A suspected case of endrin toxicosis in a cat. Vet Hum Toxicol, **27**(2): 111.

Corneliussen PE (1969) Pesticide residues in total diet samples (IV). Pestic Monit J, **2**(4): 140–152.

Corneliussen PE (1970) Pesticide residues in total diet samples (V). Pestic Monit J, **4**(3): 89–105.

Corneliussen PE (1972) Pesticide residues in total diet samples (VI). Pestic Monit J, **5**(4): 313–330.

Cote MG, Plaa GL, Valli VE, & Villeneuve DC (1985) Subchronic effects of a mixture of 'persistent' chemicals found in the Great Lakes. Bull Environ Contam Toxicol, **34**: 285–290.

Crockett AB, Wiersma GB, Tai H, & Mitchell W (1975) Pesticide and mercury residues in commercially grown catfish. Pestic Monit J, **8**(4): 235–240.

Cromartie E, Reichel WL, Locke LN, Belisle AA, Kaiser TE, Lamont TG, Mulhern BM, Prouty RM, & Swineford DM (1975) Residues of organochlorine pesticides and polychlorinated biphenyls and autopsy data for bald eagles, 1971-72. Pestic Monit J, **9**(1): 11–14.

Cueto C Jr & Biros FJ (1967) Chlorinated insecticides and related materials in human urine. Toxicol Appl Pharmacol, **10**: 261–269.

Cueto C Jr & Hayes WJ Jr (1962) The detection of dieldrin metabolites in human urine. Agric Food Chem, **10**(5): 366–369.

References

Cummings JG (1965) Pesticide residues in the total diet samples. J Assoc Off Anal Chem, **48**(6): 1177–1180.

Cummings JG (1966) Pesticides in the total diet. Residue Rev, **16**: 30–45.

Curley A, Jennings RW, Mann HT, & Sedlak V (1970) Measurement of endrin following epidemics of poisoning. Bull Environ Contam Toxicol, **5**(1): 24–29.

Currie RA, Kadis VW, Breitkreitz WE, Cunnignham GB, & Bruns GW (1979) Pesticide residues in human milk, Alberta, Canada—1966-70, 1977-78. Pestic Monit J, **13**(2): 52–55.

Dale WE, Copeland F, & Hayes WJ Jr (1965) Chlorinated insecticides in the body fat of people in India. Bull World Health Organ, **33**: 471–477.

Datta SK & Ghose KC (1985) Toxic effect of endrin on the hepatopancreas of a teleost, *Cyprinus carpio*. Indian Biol, **17**(1): 37–41.

Davies K (1988) Concentrations and dietary intake of selected organochlorines, including PCBs, PCDDs and PCDFs in fresh food composites grown in Ontario, Canada. Chemosphere, **17**(2): 263–276.

Davis GM & Lewis I (1956) Outbreak of food poisoning from bread made of chemically contaminated flour. Br Med J, **ii**: 393–398.

Davis HC & Hidu H (1969) Effects of pesticides on embryonic development of clams and oysters and on survival and growth of the larvae. Fish Bull, **67**(2): 393–404.

Dean BJ (1977) Chromosome studies on workers employed in an endrin manufacturing plant. Unpublished report No. TLGR.0008.77, Sittingbourne, Kent, Shell Research, submitted to WHO by Shell.

De Boer J (1989) Organochlorine compounds and bromodiphenylethers in livers of Atlantic cod (*Gadus morhua*) from the North Sea, 1977-1987. Chemosphere,, **18**(11/12): 2131–2140.

De Campos M & Olszyna-Marzys AE (1979) Contamination of human milk with chlorinated pesticides in Guatemala and El Salvador. Arch Environ Contam Toxicol, **8**: 43–58.

Deichmann WB & MacDonald WE (1971) Organochlorine pesticides and human health. Food Cosmet Toxicol, **9**(1): 91–103.

Deichmann WB, MacDonald WE, Blum E, Bevilacqua M, Radomski J, Keplinger M, & Balkus M (1970a) Tumorigenicity of aldrin, dieldrin and endrin in the albino rat. Ind Med, **39**(10): 426–434.

Deichmann WB, MacDonald WE, Radomski J, Blum E, Bevilacqua M, & Keplinger M (1970b) The tumorigenicity of aldrin, dieldrin, and endrin in the albino rat. Ind Med, **39**(7): 314.

Denison MS & Yarbrough JD (1985) Binding of insecticides to serum proteins in mosquitofish (*Gambusia affinis*). Comp Biochem Physiol, **81C**(1): 105–107.

Denison MS, Chambers JE, & Yarbrough JD (1985) Short-term interactions between DDT and endrin accumulation and elimination in mosquitofish (*Gambusia affinis*). Arch Environ Contam Toxicol, **14**: 315–320.

De Paula Carvalho JP, Niskikawa AM, Aranha S, & Fay EF (1984) [Organochlorine pesticide residues in bovine fat.] Biol Sao Paulo, **50**(2): 39–48 (in Portuguese).

Devault DS (1985) Contaminants in fish from Great Lakes harbors and tributary mouths. Arch Environ Contam Toxicol, **14**: 587–594.

Devault DS, Clark JM, & Lahvis G (1988) Contaminants and trends in fall run coho salmon. J Great Lakes Res, **14**(1): 23–33.

De Vos RH, van Dokkum W, Olthof PDA, Quiryns JK, Muys T, & van der Poll JM (1984) Pesticides and other chemical residues in Dutch total diet samples (June 1976-July 1978). Food Chem Toxicol **22**(1): 11-21.

Deweese LR, Cohen RR, & Stafford CJ (1985) Organochlorine residues and egg shell measurements for tree swallows *Tachycineta bicolor* in Colorado. Bull Environ Contam Toxicol, **35**: 767–775.

Dewitt JB (1965) Chronic toxicity to quail and pheasants of some chlorinated insecticides. J Agric Food Chem, **4**(10): 863–866.

Dikshith TSS & Datta KK (1973) Endrin-induced cytological changes in albino rats. Bull Environ Contam Toxicol, **9**(2): 65–69.

Dikshith TSS, Kumar SN, Raizada RB, & Srivastava MK (1989a) Organochlorine insecticide residues in cattle feed. Bull Environ Contam Toxicol, **43**: 691–696.

Dikshith TSS, Kumar SN, Tandon GS, Raizada RB, & Ray PK (1989b) Pesticide residues in edible oils and oil seeds. Bull Environ Contam Toxicol, **42**: 50–56.

Dinnel PA, Link JM, Stober QJ, Letourneau MW, & Roberts WE (1989) Comparative sensitivity of sea urchin sperm bioassays to metals and pesticides. Arch Environ Contam Toxicol, **18**: 748–755.

Ditraglia D, Brown DP, Namekata T, & Iverson N (1981) Mortality study of workers employed at organochlorine pesticide manufacturing plants. Scand J Work Environ Health, **7**(suppl 4): 140–146.

References

Donahue JF, Burse VW, Head SL, & Andrews JS (1988) Comparison of two techniques for quantifying environmental contaminants in human serum. Life Sci, 43: 2257–2264.

Donoso J, Dorigan J, Fuller B, Gordon J, Kornreich M, Saari S, Thomas L, & Walker P (1979) Reviews of the environmental effects of pollutants. XIII. Endrin. Oak Ridge, Tennessee, Oak Ridge National Laboratory (EPA-600/1-79-005).

DouAbul AAZ, Al-Saad HT, Al-Obaidy SZ, & Al-Rekabi HN (1987a) Residues of organochlorine pesticides in fish from the Arabian Gulf. Water Air Soil Pollut, 35: 187–194.

DouAbul AAZ, Al-Saad HT, & Al-Rekabi HN (1987b) Residues of organochlorine pesticides in environmental samples from the Shatt al-Arab River, Iraq. Environ Pollut, 43: 175–187.

DouAbul AAZ, Al-Omar M, Al-Obaidy S, & Al-Ogaily N (1987c) Organochlorine pesticide residues in fish from the Shatt al-Arab River, Iraq. Bull Environ Contam Toxicol, 38: 674–680.

DouAbul AAZ, Al-Saad HT, Al-Timari AA, & Al-Rekabi HN (1988) Tigris-Euphrates delta: a major source of pesticides to the Shatt al-Arab River (Iraq). Arch Environ Contam Toxicol, 17: 405–418.

Dowd PF, Mayfield GU, Coulon DP, Graves JB, & Newsom JD (1985) Organochlorine residues in animals from three Louisiana watersheds in 1978 and 1979. Bull Environ Contam Toxicol, 34: 832–841.

Duggan RE & Corneliussen PE (1972) Dietary intake of pesticide chemicals in the United States (III), June 1968-1970. Pestic Monit J, 5(4): 331–341.

Duggan RE & Lipscomb GQ (1969) Dietary intake of pesticide chemicals in the United States (II), June 1966-April 1968. Pestic Monit J, 2(4): 153–162.

Duggan RE, Barry HC, & Johnson LY (1966) Pesticide residues in total diet samples. Science, 151: 101–104.

Duggan RE, Barry HC, & Johnson LY (1967) Pesticide residues in total diet samples (II). Pestic Monit J, 1(2): 2–12.

Duke TW & Dumas DP (1974) Implications of pesticide residues in the coastal environment. In: Vernberg FJ & Vernberg WB, ed. Pollution and physiology of marine organisms. New York, Academic Press, pp 137–164.

Dureja P, Walia S, & Mukerjee SK (1987) New photometabolites of endrin. Indian J Chem, 26G: 898–899.

Durham WF & Wolfe HR (1962) Measurement of the exposure of workers to pesticides. Bull World Health Organ, 26: 75–91.

Dutch Agricultural Advisory Commission on Environmental Pollutants (1983) Annual report. The Hague, Ministry of Agriculture, Management of Nature and Fisheries.

Earnest RD & Benville PE Jr (1972) Acute toxicity of four organochlorine insecticides to two species of surf perch. California Fish Game, 58(2): 127–132.

Egan H, Goulding R, Roburn J, & Tatton JO'G (1965) Organochlorine pesticide residues in human fat and human milk. Br Med J, ii: 66.

Eisenberg M & Topping JJ (1985) Organochlorine residues in finfish from Maryland waters 1976-1980. J Environ Sci Health B20(6): 729-742.

Eisler R (1970a) Latent effects of insecticide intoxication to marine molluscs. Hydrobiologia, 36(3-4): 345–352.

Eisler R (1970b) Acute toxicities of organochlorine and organophosphorus insecticides to estuarine fish. Tech Paper Bur Sport Fish Wildl, 46: 1–12.

El-Dib MA & Badawy MI (1985) Organochlorine insecticides and PCB's in river Nile water, Egypt. Bull Environ Contam Toxicol, 34: 126–133.

Ellis DH, Deweese LR, Grubb TG, Kiff LF, Smith DG, Jarman WM, & Peakall DB (1989) Pesticide residues in Arizona peregrine falcon eggs and prey. Bull Environ Contam Toxicol, 42: 57–64.

Elnabarawy MT, Welter AN, & Robideau RR (1986) Relative sensitivity of three daphnid species to selected organic and inorganic chemicals. Environ Toxicol Chem, 5: 393–398.

El Nabawi A, Heinzow B, & Kruse H (1987) Residue levels of organochlorine chemicals and polychlorinated biphenyls in fish from the Alexandria Region, Egypt. Arch Environ Contam Toxicol, 16: 689–696.

El-Sebae AH (1987) Acute and chronic toxicity to marine biota of widely used dispersants, PCBs, chlorinated pesticides and their combinations and their biomagnification in Alexandria region. In: Research on the toxicity, persistence, bioaccumulation, carcinogenicity and mutagenicity of selected substances (Activity G). Final reports on projects dealing with toxicity (1983–1985). Athens, United Nations Environment Programme (Mediterranean Action Plan (MAP), Technical Reports Series No. 10).

Ely RE, Moore LA, Carter RH, & App BA (1957) Excretion of endrin in the milk of cows fed endrin-sprayed alfalfa and technical endrin. J Econ Entomol, 50(3): 348–349.

Emerson TE Jr (1965) Mechanisms of hemoconcentration in the dog during acute endrin insecticide poisoning. Can J Physiol Pharmacol, 43: 793–800.

Emerson TE Jr & Hinshaw LB (1965) Peripheral vascular effects of the insecticide endrin. Can J Physiol Pharmacol, 43: 531–539.

References

Emerson TE Jr, Brake CM, & Hinshaw LB (1963) Mechanism of Action of the Insecticide Endrin. Oklahoma City, Oklahoma, Civil Aeromedical Research Institute (Report No. 63-16).

Emerson TE Jr, Brake CM, & Hinshaw LB (1964) Cardiovascular effects of the insecticide endrin. Can J Physiol Pharmacol, **42**: 41–51.

Engst R & Knoll R (1973) [On the contamination of surface, rain and drinking waters with chlorinated hydrocarbons.] Nahrung, **17**(8): 837–851 (in German with English summary).

Epstein SS, Arnold E, Andrea J, Bass W, & Bishop Y (1972) Detection of chemical mutagens by the dominant lethal assay in the mouse. Toxicol Appl Pharmacol, **23**: 288–325.

Ercegovich CD & Rashid KA (1977) Mutagenesis induced in mutant strains of *Salmonella typhimurium* by pesticides. In: Abstracts of the 174th ACS National Meeting, Chicago, Illinois. Washington, DC, American Chemical Society, Division of Pesticide Chemistry (Abstract No. 43).

Everaarts JM, Koeman JH, & Brader, L (1971) Contribution à l'étude des effets sur quelques éléments de la faune sauvage des insecticides organo-chlorés utilisés au Tchad en culture cotonnière. Cotton Fibre Trop, **26**(4): 385–394.

Fabacher DL & Chambers H (1976) Uptake and storage of ^{14}C-labelled endrin by the livers and brains of pesticide-susceptible and resistant mosquitofish. Bull Environ Contam Toxicol, **16**(2): 203–207.

Fahrig R (1974) Comparative mutagenicity studies with pesticides. In: Montesano R & Tomatis L ed. Chemical carcinogenesis essays. Lyon, International Agency for Research on Cancer, pp 161–181 (IARC Scientific Publications No. 10).

FAO (1982) Second Government Consultation on International Harmonization of Pesticide Registration Requirements, Rome, 11–15 October 1982. Rome, Food and Agriculture Organization of the United Nations.

FAO/WHO (1964) Evaluation of the toxicity of pesticide residues in food. Report of a joint meeting of the FAO Committee on Pesticides in Agriculture and the WHO Expert Committee on Pesticide Residues, Geneva, World Health Organization (FAO Meeting Report No. PL:1963/13; WHO/Food Add./23).

FAO/WHO (1965) Evaluation of the toxicity of pesticide residues in food. Geneva, World Health Organization (FAO Meeting Report No. PL:1965/10/1; WHO/Food Add./27.65).

FAO/WHO (1971) Joint meeting of FAO Working Party of Experts and the WHO Expert Group on Pesticide Residues. 1970 Evaluation of some pesticide residues in food. Geneva, World Health Organization (AGP:1979/M/12/1; WHO Food Add./71.42).

FAO/WHO (1984) Codex guidelines on good practice in pesticide residue analysis. Rome, Codex Alimentarius Commission, Food and Agriculture Organization of the United Nations (CAC/PR7-1984).

FAO/WHO (1986a) Recommendations for methods of analysis of pesticide residues. Rome, Codex Alimentarius Commission, Food and Agriculture Organization of the United Nations (CAC/PR8-1986).

FAO/WHO (1986b) Codex maximum limits for pesticide residues. Rome, Codex Alimentarius Commission, Joint FAO/WHO Food Standards Programme, Food and Agriculture Organization of the United Nations, p 33-IV (FAO CAC Vol. XIII, ed. 2).

Fasola M, Vecchio I, Caccialanza G, Gandini C, & Kitsos M (1987) Trends of organochlorine residues in eggs of birds from Italy, 1977 to 1985. Environ Pollut, **48**: 25–36.

FDA (1988) Food and Drug Administration pesticide program. Residues in foods—1987. J Assoc Off Anal Chem, **71**(6): 156A–174A.

Ferguson DE, Culley DD, & Cotton WD (1964) Resistance to chlorinated hydrocarbon insecticides in three species of freshwater fish. Bioscience, **14**: 43–44.

Flickinger EL & King KA (1972) Some effects of aldrin-treated rice on Gulf Coast wildlife. J Wildl Manage, **36**: 706–727.

Flickinger EL, Mitchell CA, & Krynitsky AJ (1986) Dieldrin and endrin residues in fulvous whistling ducks in Texas in 1983. J. Field Ornithol, **57**(2): 85–192.

Folmar LC (1978) *In vitro* inhibition of rat brain ATPase, pNPPase, and ATP-^{32}Pi exchange by chlorinated-diphenyl ethanes and cyclodiene insecticides. Bull Environ Contam Toxicol, **19**: 481–488.

Foschi F, Natali G, Guberti MG, Camisani MG, Taccheto Barbina M, Spessotto C, & Bargarolo L (1985) [Study on residues of argicultural chemicals in apples.] Inf Fitopatol, **12**: 14–20 (in Italian).

Fournier E, Treich I, Campagne L, & Capelle N (1972) Pesticides organo-chlorés dans le tissu adipeux d'êtres humains en France. Eur J Toxicol, **1**(1): 11–26.

Fox ME, Roper DS, & Thrush SF (1988) Organochlorine contaminants in surficial sediments of Manukau Harbour, New Zealand. Mar Pollut Bull,**19**(7): 333–336.

Frank R, Braun HE, Holdrinet M, Sirons GJ, Smith EH, & Dixon DW (1979) Organochlorine insecticides and industrial pollutants in the milk supply of Southern Ontario, Cananda—1977. J Food Prot, **42**(1): 31–37.

References

Frank R, Braun HE, & Holdrinet MVH (1981) Residues from past uses of organochlorine pesticides and PCB in waters draining eleven agricultural watersheds in Southern Ontario, Canada, 1975-1977. Sci Total Environ, 20: 255–276.

Frank R, Braun HE, Sirons GH, Rasper J, & Ward GG (1985) Organochlorine and organophosphorus insecticides and industrial pollutants in the milk supplies of Ontario— 1983. J Food Prot, 48(6): 499–504.

Fredrickson DS (1978) Report on bioassay of endrin for possible carcinogenicity. Fed Reg, 43(225): 54298.

Gaines TB (1960) The acute toxicity of pesticides to rats. Toxicol Appl Pharmacol, 2: 88–99.

Gaines TB (1969) Acute toxicity of pesticides. Toxicol Appl Pharmacol, 14: 515–534.

Galassi S & Provini A (1981) Chlorinated pesticides and PCBs contents of the two main tributaries into the Adriatic Sea. Sci Total Environ, 17: 51–57.

Gant DB, Eldefrawi ME, & Eldefrawi AT (1987) Cyclodiene insecticides inhibit GABAa receptor-regulated chloride transport. Toxicol Appl Pharmacol, 88(3): 313–321.

Garrett NE, Stack HF, & Waters MD (1986) Evaluation of the genetic activity profiles of 65 pesticides. Mutat Res, 168(3): 301–325.

Gartrell MJ, Craun JC, Podrebarac DS, & Gunderson EL (1986a) Pesticides, selected elements, and other chemicals in adult total diet samples October 1980-March 1982. J Assoc Off Anal Chem, 69(1): 146–161.

Gartrell MJ, Craun JC, Podrebarac DS, & Gunderson EL (1986b) Pesticides, selected elements, and other chemicals in infant and toddler total diet samples, October 1980-March 1982. J Assoc Off Anal Chem, 69(1): 123–145.

Giesy JP, Mewsted J, & Garling DL (1986) Relationships between chlorinated hydrocarbon concentrations and rearing mortality of chinook salmon (*Onchorhynchus tshawytscha*) eggs from Lake Michigan. J Great Lakes Res, 12(1): 82–98.

Gips T (1987) Breaking the pesticide habit—Alternatives to 12 hazardous pesticides (International Alliance for Sustainable Agriculture (IASA) Publication No. 1987-2).

Glatt H, Jung R, & Oesch F (1983) Bacterial mutagenicity investigation of epoxides: drugs, drug metabolites, steroids and pesticides. Mutat Res, 11: 99–118.

Glooschenko WA, Strachan WMJ, & Sampson RCJ (1976) Distribution of pesticides and polychlorinated biphenyls in water, sediments and seston of the Upper Great Lakes— 1974. Pestic Monit J, 10(2): 61–67.

Gluth G & Hanke W (1985) A comparison of physiological changes in carp, *Cyprinus carpio*, induced by several pollutants at sub-lethal concentrations. I. The dependency on exposure time. Ecotoxicol Environ Saf, **9**: 179–188.

Godsil PJ & Johnson WC (1968) Pesticide monitoring of the aquatic biota of the Tule Lake National Wildlife Refuge. Pestic Monit J, **1**(4): 21–26.

Goerlitz DF & Law LM (1974) Determination of chlorinated insecticides in suspended sediment and bottom material. J Assoc Off Anal Chem, **57**(1): 176–181.

Goldentahl El (1978a) Teratology study in rats. Unpublished report No. 163-488, International Research and Development Corporation, submitted to WHO by Shell.

Goldentahl El (1978b) Teratology study in hamsters. Unpublished report No. 163-478, International Research and Development Corporation, submitted to WHO by Shell.

Good EE & Ware GW (1969) Effects of insecticides on reproduction in the laboratory mouse. Toxicol Appl Pharmacol, **14**: 201–203.

Graves JB & Bradley JR (1965) Response of Swiss albino mice to intraperitoneal injection of endrin. J Econ Entomol, **58**(1): 178–179.

Gray LE Jr, Kavlock RJ, Chernoff N, Gray JA, & McLamb J (1981) Perinatal toxicity of endrin in rodents. III. Alterations of behavioural ontogeny. Toxicology, **21**: 187–202.

Green DR, Stull JK, & Heesen TC (1986) Determination of chlorinated hydrocarbons in coastal waters using a moored *in situ* sampler and transported live mussels. Mar Pollut Bull, **17**(7): 324–329.

Gregor DJ & Gummer WD (1989) Evidence of atmospheric transport and deposition of organochlorine pesticides and polychlorinated biphenyls in Canadian Arctic snow. Environ Sci Technol, **23**: 561–565.

Gübeli T & Clerc JT (1988) [Detection of pesticide residues in ethanol extracts of plants.] Pharm Acta Helv, **63**(3): 85–89 (in German).

Guicherit R & Schulting FL (1985) The occurrence of organic chemicals in the atmosphere of the Netherlands. Sci Total Environ, **43**: 193–219.

Gunderson EL (1988) FDA total diet study, April 1982-April 1984, dietary intakes of pesticides, selected elements and other chemicals. J Assoc Off Anal Chem, **71**(6): 1200–1209.

Hall RJ & Swineford D (1980) Toxic effects of endrin and toxaphene on the southern leopard frog *Rana sphenocephala*. In: Mellanby, K. ed. Environmental pollution. Barking, Essex, Applied Science Publishing, pp 53–65.

References

Hall LW Jr, Hall WS, Bushong SJ, & Herman RL (1987) In situ striped bass (*Morone saxatilis*) contaminant and water quality studies in the Potomac River. Aquat Toxicol, **10**: 73–99.

Hamdy Y & Post L (1985) Distribution of mercury, trace organics and other heavy metals in Detroit River sediments. J Great Lakes Res, **11**(3): 353–365.

Hansen DJ, Schimmel SC, & Forester J (1977) Endrin: effects on the entire life cycle of a saltwater fish, *Cyprinodon variegatus*. J Toxicol Environ Health, **3**: 721–733.

Harris CR, Sans WW, & Miles JRW (1966) Exploratory studies on the occurrence of organochlorine insecticides residues in agricultural soils in southwestern Ontario. J Agric Food Chem,**14**(4): 398–403.

Hart LG & Fouts JR (1963) Effects of acute and chronic DDT administration in hepatic microsomal drug metabolism in the rat (28686). Proc Soc Exp Biol Med,**114**: 388–392.

Hartgrove RW Jr, Hundley SG, & Webb RE (1977) Characterization of the hepatic mixed function oxidase system in endrin resistant and -suspectible pinevoles. Pestic Biochem Physiol, **7**(2): 146–153.

Hashemy-Tonkabony SE & Mosstofian B (1979) Chlorinated pesticide residues in chicken egg. Poult Sci **58**(6): 1432-1434.

Hashemy-Tonkabony SE & Soleimani-Amiri MJ (1976) Detection and determination of chlorinated pesticide residues in raw and various stages of processed vegetable oil. J Am Oil Chem Soc, **53**(12): 752–753.

Hashimoto I & Nishiuchi S (1981) Establishment of bioassay methods for evaluation of acute toxicity of pesticides to aquatic organisms. J Pestic Sci, **6**: 257–264.

Hassett AJ, Viljoen PT, & Liebenberg JJE (1987) An assessment of chlorinated pesticides in the major surface water resources of the Orange Free State during the period September 1984 to September 1985.Water SA, **13**(3): 133–136.

Hawker DW & Connell DW (1986) Bioconcentration of lipophilic compounds by some aquatic organisms. Ecotoxicol Environ Saf, **11**: 184–197.

Hawthorne JC, Ford JH, & Markin GP (1974) Residues of mirex and other chlorinated pesticides in commercially raised catfish. Bull Environ Contam Toxicol, **11**(3): 258–264.

Hayes WJ Jr (1963) Clinical handbook on economic poisons. Emergency information for treating poisoning. Atlanta, Georgia, US Department of Health, Education, and Welfare, Communicable Disease Center, Toxicology Section, pp 68–70.

Hayes WJ Jr (1975) Toxicology of pesticides, Baltimore, Maryland,Williams & Wilkins, pp 288–294.

Hayes WJ Jr (1982) Pesticides studied in man, Baltimore, Maryland, Williams and Wilkins, pp 247–251.

Hayes WJ Jr & Curley A (1968) Storage and excretion of dieldrin and related compounds. Effect of occupational exposure. Arch Environ Health, **16**(2): 155–162.

Hayes WJ Jr, Dale WE, & Burse VW (1965) Chlorinated hydrocarbon pesticides in the fat of people in New Orleans. Life Sci, **4**: 1611–1615.

Heidmann WA, Büthe A, Beyerbach M, Löhmer R, & Rüssel-Sinn HA (1989) [Chlorinated hydrocarbons of some bird species breeding in the inland of Lower Saxony.] J Ornitol, **130**(3): 311–320 (in German with English summary).

Heinz GH, Erdman TC, Haseltine SD, & Stafford C (1985) Contaminant levels in colonial waterbirds from Green Bay and Lake Michigan, 1975–80. Environ Monit Assess, **5**: 223–236.

Henderson C, Johnson WL, & Inglis A (1969) Organochlorine insecticide residues in fish. National pesticides monitoring program. Pestic Monit J, **3**: 145–171.

Henderson C, Inglis A, & Johnson WL (1971) Organochlorine insecticide residues in fish. Fall 1969, National Pesticide Monitoring Program. Pestic Monit J, **5**: 1–11.

Hendrickson CM & Bowden JA (1976) In vitro inhibition of lactic acid dehydrogenase by insecticidal polychlorinated hydrocarbons. 2. Inhibition by dieldrin and related compounds. J Agric Food Chem, **24**(4): 756–759.

Hendrickx A & Maes R (1969) The excretion of chlorinated hydrocarbon insecticides in human mother milk. J Pharm Belg, **24**(9–10): 459–463.

Hermanutz R (1974) Quarterly report. Duluth, Minnesota, US Environmental Protection Agency, National Water Quality Laboratory.

Hermanutz RO, Eaton JG, & Mueller LH (1985) Toxicity of endrin and malathion mixtures to flagfish (*Jordanella floridae*). Arch Environ Contam Toxicol, **14**: 307–314.

Hernandez FH, Lopez Benet FJ, Escriche JM, & Ubeda JCB (1987) Sulfuric acid cleanup and KOH-ethanol treatment for confirmation of organochlorine pesticides and polychlorinated biphenyls: application to wastewater samples. J Assoc Off Anal Chem, **70**(4): 727–733.

Herrera Marteache A, Polo Villar LM, Jodral Villarejo M, Polo Villar G, Mallol J, & Pozo Lora R (1978) [Organochlorine pesticide residues in human fat in Spain.] Rev San Hig Publico, **52**: 1125–1144 (in Spanish with English summary).

Hill EF & Camardese MB (1986) Lethal dietary toxicities of environmental contaminants and pesticides to Coturnix. Washington, DC, US Department of the Interior, Fish and Wildlife Service, p 147 (Fish and Wildlife Technical Report No. 2).

References

Hill EF, Health RG, Spann JW, & Williams JD (1975) Lethal dietary toxicities of environmental pollutants to birds. Washington, DC, US Department of the Interior, Fish and Wildlife Service (Special Scientific Report: Wildlife No. 191).

Hill RH Jr, Needham LL, & Liddle JA (1986) The laboratory's role in environmental health emergency investigations. Clin Toxicol, **24**(5): 363–374.

Hine CH (1965) Results of reproduction study of rats fed diets containing endrin insecticide over three generations. Unpublished report No. 2, San Francisco, CA, Hine Laboratories, submitted to WHO by Shell.

Hine CH (1968) Results of reproduction study of rats fed diets containing endrin insecticide over three generations. Unpublished report No. 7, San Francisco, CA, Hine Laboratories, submitted to WHO by Shell.

Hine CH, Anderson HH, Kodama JK, & Gutenberg EF (1954) Class B evaluation of endrin compositions. Unpublished report No. 223, San Francisco, CA, University of California School of Medicine, submitted to WHO by Shell.

Hinshaw LB, Solomon LA, Reins DA, Fiorica V, & Emerson TE (1966) Effects of the insecticide endrin on the cardiovascular system of the dog. J Pharmacol Exp Ther, **153**(2): 225–236.

Hirom PC, Millburn P, Smith RL, & Williams RT (1972) Species variations in the threshold molecular-weight factor for the biliary excretion of organic anions. Biochem J, **129**: 1071–1077.

Hoffman WS, Fishbein WI, & Andelman MB (1964) The pesticide content of human fat tissue. Arch Environ Health, **9**: 387–394.

Hoffman WS, Adler H, Fishbein WI, & Bauer FC (1967) Relation of pesticide concentration in fat to pathological changes in tissues. Arch Environ Health, **15**: 758–765.

Hogmire HW, Weaver JE, & Brooks JL (1990) Survey for pesticides in wells associated with apple and peach orchards in West Virginia. Bull Environ Contam Toxicol, **44**: 81–86.

Holden AV (1970) International cooperative study of organo-chlorine pesticide residues in terrestrial and aquatic wildlife, 1967/1968. Pestic Monit J, **4**(3): 117–135.

Hoogendam I, Versteeg JPJ, & de Vlieger M (1962) Electroencephalograms in insecticide toxicity. Arch Environ Health, **4**: 86–94.

Hoogendam I, Versteeg JPJ, & de Vlieger M (1965) Nine years toxicity control in insecticide plants. Arch Environ Health, **10**: 441–448.

Horn H, Hartner L, & von Faber H (1987) [On the suitability of liver function tests in birds for the ecotoxicological evaluation of environmental chemicals.] Dtsch Tierarztl Wochenschr, **94**: 1–48 (in German with English summary).

Horsfall F Jr, Webb RE, Price NO, & Young RW (1970) Residues in apples subsequent to ground sprays of endrin. J Agric Food Chem, **18**: 221–223.

Hrdina PD, Singhal RL, & Peters DAV (1974) Changes in brain biogenic amines and body temperature after cyclodiene insecticides. Toxicol Appl Pharmacol, **29**(1): 119.

Hrubec J (1988) [Pesticides and drinking-water.] H_2O, **21**(11): 278–282 (in Dutch).

Hudson RH, Tucker RK, & Haegele MA (1984) Handbook of toxicity of pesticides to wildlife. Washington, DC, US Department of the Interior, Fish and Wildlife Service (Resource Publication 153).

Hunter CG, Robinson J, & Richardson A (1963) Chlorinated insecticide content of human body fat in southern England. Br Med J, **i**: 221–224.

Hunter J, Maxwell JD, Carrella M, Stewart DW, & Williams R (1971) Urinary-D-glucaric acid excretion as a test for hepatic enzyme induction in man. Lancet, **20 March**: 572–575.

Hunter J, Maxwell JD, Stewart DW, Williams R, Robinson J, & Richardson A (1972) Increased hepatic microsomal enzymes activity from occupational exposure to certain organochlorine pesticides. Nature, **237**: 399–401.

Hutson DH (1981) The metabolism of insecticides in man. In: Hutson DH & Roberts TR ed. Progress in pesticide biochemistry. New York, John Wiley and Sons, vol 1, pp 287–333.

Hutson DH & Hoadley EC (1974) The oxidation of a cyclic alcohol (12-hydroxyendrin) to a ketone (12-ketoendrin) by microsomal mono-oxygenation. Chemosphere, **5**: 205–210.

Hutson DH, Baldwin MK, & Hoadley EC (1975) Detoxication and bioactivation of endrin in the rat. Xenobiotica, **5**(11): 697–714.

IARC (1974) Endrin. In: Some organochlorine pesticides. Lyon, International Agency for Research on Cancer, pp. 157–171 (IARC Monographs on the Evaluation of Carcinogenic Risk of Chemicals to Man, Volume 5).

IARC (1987) Overall evaluations of carcinogenicity: An updating of IARC Monographs volumes 1 to 42. Lyon, International Agency for Research on Cancer, p. 63 (IARC Monographs on the Evaluation of Carcinogenic Risks to Humans, Supplement 7).

Illahi A, Amin N, Hashmi AS, Nawaz M, & Naeem-ur Rahman (1986) Incidence of endrin residues in cucumber and its effects on the biological system of rats. J Pak Med Assoc, **36**(8): 209–211.

References

Illahi A, Roohi J, & Hashmi AS (1987) Present status of endrin residues in peas and its effect on biological systems. J Pure Appl Sci, **6**(1): 1–4.

Ito N, Tatematsu M, Nakanishi K, Hasegawa R, Takano T, Imaida K, & Ogiso T (1980) The effects of various chemicals on the development of hyperplastic liver nodules in hepatectomized rats treated with N-nitrosodimethylamine or N-2-fluorenylacetamide. Gann, **71**: 832–842.

Jacobziner H & Raybin HW (1959) Briefs on accidental chemical poisonings in New York City. Poisoning by insecticide (endrin). NY State J Med, **59**: 2017–2022.

Jager KW (1970) Aldrin, dieldrin, endrin and telodrin. An epidemiological study of long-term occupational exposure. Amsterdam, Elsevier Science Publishers.

Japanese Environmental Agency (1975) Environmental survey report on chemical substances in FY 1974. Unpublished report, December 1975, Tokyo, Environmental Health Department, Planning and Coordination Bureau.

Japenga J, Wagenaar WJ, Smedes F, & Salomons W (1987) A new, rapid clean-up procedure for the simultaneous determination of different groups of organic micropollutants in sediments; application in two European estuarine sediment studies. Environ Technol Lett, **8**(1): 9–20.

Jarvinen AW, Tanner DK, & Kline ER (1988) Toxicity of chlorpyrifos, endrin, or fenvalerate to fathead minnows following episodic or continuous exposure. Ecotoxicol Environ Saf, **15**: 78–95.

Jedeikin R, Kaplan R, Shapira A, Radwan H, & Hoffman S (1979) The successful use of 'high level' PEEP in near fatal endrin poisoning. Crit Care Med, **7**(4): 168–170.

Jegier Z (1964) Health hazards in insecticide spraying of crops. Arch Environ Health, **8**: 670–674.

Jenkins RB & Toole JF (1964) Polyneuropathy following exposure to insecticides. Arch Intern Med, **113**: 691–695.

Johnson DW (1968) Pesticides and fishes—a review of selected literature. Trans Am Fish Soc, **97**(4) 398–424.

Johnson RD & Manske DD (1976) Pesticide residues in total diet samples (IX). Pestic Monit J, **9**(4): 157–169.

Johnson RD & Manske DD (1977) Pesticide and other chemical residues in total diet samples (XI). Pestic Monit J, **11**(3): 116–131.

Johnson RD, Manske DD, New DH, & Podrebarac DS (1979) Pesticide and other chemical residues in infant and toddler total diet samples, (I), August 1974-July 1975. Pestic Monit J, **13**(3): 87–98.

Johnson RD, Manske DD, & Podrebarac DS (1981a) Pesticide, metal, and other chemical residues in adult total diet samples, (XII), August 1975-July 1976. Pestic Monit J, **15**(1): 54–71.

Johnson RD, Manske DD, New DH, & Podrebarac DS (1981b) Pesticide, heavy metal, and other chemical residues in infant and toddler total diet samples, (II), August 1975-July 1976. Pestic Monit J, **15**(1): 39–50.

Johnson RD, Manske DD, New DH, & Podrebarac DS (1984) Pesticide, metal, and other chemical residues in adult total diet samples, (XIII), August 1976-July 1977. J Assoc Off Anal Chem, **67**(1): 154–166.

Johnson MG, Kelso JRM, & George SE (1988) Loadings of organochlorine contaminants and trace elements to two Ontario lake systems and their concentrations in fish. Can J Fish Aquat Sci, **45**: 170–178.

Jolley WP, Stemmer KL, Grande F, Richmon J, & Pfitzer EA (1969) The effects exerted upon beagle dogs during a period of two years by the introduction of 1,2,3,4,10,10-hexachloro-6,7-epoxy-1,4,4a,5,6,7,8,8a-octahydro-1,4-endo,endo-5,8-dimethanonaphthalene into their daily diets. Unpublished report, Cincinnati, Ohio, Kettering Laboratory, submitted to WHO by Shell.

Joy RM (1976) Convulsive properties of chlorinated hydrocarbon insecticides in the cat central nervous system. Toxicol Appl Pharmacol, **35**: 95–106.

Kacew S, Sutherland DJB, & Singhal RL (1973) Biochemical changes following chronic administration of heptachlor, heptachlor epoxide and endrin to male rats. Environ Physiol Biochem, **3**: 221–229.

Kachole MS & Pawar SS (1977) Effect of endrin on microsomal electron transport reactions. Part I: Sleeping time, electron transport components and protection due to pretreatments. Abstracts of the 1976 Annual General Meeting of Biochemists. J Biochem, **14**(1): 45.

Kadis VW, Breitkreitz WE, & Jonasson OJ (1970) Insecticide levels in human tissues of Alberta residents. Can J Public Health, **61**(5): 413–416.

Kagan J, Kagan ED, & Seigneurie E (1986) Alpha-terthienyl, a powerful fish poison with light-dependent activity. Chemosphere, **15**(1): 49–57.

Kaiser TE, Reichel WL, Locke LN, Cromartie E, Lamont TG, Mulhern BM, Prouty RM, Stafford CJ, & Swineford DM (1980) Organochlorine pesticide, PCB, PBB residues and necropsy data for bald eagles from 29 states—1975-77. Pestic Monit J, **13**: 145–149.

Kampe W (1985) [Pesticide residues in animal feeding-stuffs.] Dtsch Tierarztl Wochenschr, **92**(6): 228–231 (in German).

References

Kanitz S & Castello G (1966) [The presence of residues of some pesticides in human fatty tissue and in some foods. Initial results of a survey carried out in Liguria.] G Ig Med Prev, **7**: 1–19 (in Italian).

Karplus M (1971) [Endrin poisoning in children.] Harefuah, **18**(3): 113–116 (in Hebrew with English summary).

Kassabi M, ElHraiki A, & Nader B (1988) Contamination of urban, industrial and continental waters by chlorinated hydrocarbon pesticides along the mediterranean coast of Morocco. Sci Total Environ, **71**: 209–214.

Kathpal T & Dewan RS (1975) Improved clean-up technique for the estimation of endosulfan and endrin residues. J Assoc Off Anal Chem, **58**(5): 1076–1078.

Katz M & Chadwick GG (1961) Toxicity of endrin to some Pacific Northwest fishes. Trans Am Fish Soc, **90**: 394–397.

Kavlock RJ, Chernoff N, Hanisch RC, Gray J, Rogers E, & Gray LE Jr (1981) Perinatal toxicity of endrin in rodents. II. Fetotoxic effects of prenatal exposure in rats and mice. Toxicology, **21**: 141–150.

Kavlock RJ, Chernoff N, & Rogers EH (1985) The effect of acute maternal toxicity on fetal development in the mouse. Teratog Carcinog Mutagen, **5**: 3–13.

Kavlock RJ, Rogers JM, Gray LE, & Chernoff N (1987) Postnatal alterations in development resulting from prenatal exposure to pesticides. In: Pesticide science and biotechnology, Proceedings of the 6th International Congress on Pesticide Chemicals, pp 561–564.

Keilty TJ & Stehly GR (1989) Preliminary investigation of protein utilization by an aquatic earthworm in response to sublethal stress. Bull Environ Contam Toxicol, **43**: 350–354.

Keilty TJ, White DS, & Landrum PF (1988a) Short-term lethality and sediment avoidance assays with endrin-contaminated sediment and two Oligochaetes from Lake Michigan. Arch Environ Contam Toxicol, **17**: 95–101.

Keilty TJ, White DS, & Landrum PF (1988b) Sublethal responses to endrin in sediment by *Limnodrilus hoffmeisteri* (Tubificidae) and in mixed-culture with *Stylodrilus heringianus* (Lumbriculidae). Aquat Toxicol, **13**: 227–250.

Keilty TJ, White DS, & Landrum PF (1988c) Sublethal responses to endrin in sediment by Stylodrilus heringianus (Lumbriculidae) as measured by a 137cesium marker layer technique. Aquat Toxicol, **13**: 251–270.

Keplinger MK & Deichmann WB (1967) Acute toxicity of combinations of pesticides. Toxicol Appl Pharmacol, **10**: 586–595.

Khangarot BS, Sehgal A, & Bhasin MK (1985) Man and biosphere—studies on the Sikkim Himalayas. Part 6: Toxicity of selected pesticides to frog tadpole, *Rana hexadactyla* (Lesson). Acta Hydrochim Hydrobiol, **13**(3): 391-394.

Kiang PH & Grob RL (1986) Development of a screening method for the determination of 49 priority pollutants in soil. J Environ Sci Health, **A21**(1): 15–53.

Kiene RP & Capone DG (1984) Effects of organic pollutants on methanogenesis, sulfate reduction and carbon dioxide evolution in salt marsh sediments. Mar Environ Res **13**: 141–160.

Kiigemagi U, Sprowls RG, & Terriere LC (1958) Endrin content of milk and body tissues of dairy cows receiving endrin daily in their diet. J Agric Food Chem, **6**(7): 518–521.

King KA, Flickinger EL, & Hildebrand HH (1977) The decline of brown pelicans on the Lousiana and Texas Gulf Coast. Southwest Nat, **21**(4): 417–431.

King KA, Blankinship DR, Payne E, Krynitsky AJ, & Hensler GL (1985) Brown pelican populations and pollutants in Texas, 1975-1981. Wilson Bull, **97**(2): 201–214.

Kinoshita FK & Kempf CK (1970) Quantitative measurement of hepatic microsomal enzyme induction after dietary intake of chlorinated hydrocarbon insecticides. Toxicol Appl Pharmacol, **17**: 288.

Klein W, Mueller W, & Korte F (1968) [Insecticides in the metabolism. XVI. Excretion, distribution and metabolism of endrin ^{14}C in rats.] Liebigs Ann Chem,**713**: 180–185.

Klevay LM (1971) Endrin excretion by the isolated perfused rat liver: a sexual difference. Proc Soc Exp Biol Med, **136**: 878–879.

Kodavanti PRS, Mehrotra BD, Chetty SC, & Desaiah D (1988) Effect of selected insecticides on rat brain synaptosomal adenylate cyclase and phosphodiesterase. J Toxicol Environ Health, **25**: 207–215.

Koeman JH (1971) [The occurrence and the toxicological implications of some chlorinated hydrocarbons in the Dutch coastal area in the period 1965–70], Utrecht, Rijks University, pp 88, 96 (Thesis) (in Dutch).

Koeman JH, Oskamp AAG, Veen J, Brouwer E, Rooth J, Zwart P, van de Brock E, & van Genderen H (1967) Insecticides as a factor in the mortality of the sandwich tern (*Sterna sandvicensis*). A preliminary communication. Meded Fac Landbouwwet Rijksuniv Gent, **32**: 841–854.

Koeman JH, Vink JAJ, & de Goeij JJM (1969) Causes of mortality in birds of prey and owls in the Netherlands in the winter of 1968-69. Andrea, **57**: 67–76.

Koeman JH, Pennings JH, de Goeij JJM, Tjioe PS, Olindo PM, & Hopcraft J (1972) A preliminary survey of the possible contamination of Lake Nakuru in Kenya with some metals and chlorinated hydrocarbon pesticides. J Appl Ecol, 9(2): 411–416.

Koeman JH, Pennings JH, Rosanto R, Soemarwoto O, Tjioe PS, Blancke S, Kusumadinata S, & Djajadiredja RR (1974) Metals and chlorinated hydrocarbon pesticides in samples of fish, sawah-duck eggs, crustaceans and molluscs collected in Indonesia in April and May 1972. Unpublished report, Wageningen-Bandung, University of Wageningen, The Netherlands.

Korn S & Earnest R (1974) Acute toxicity of twenty insecticides to striped bass, *Morone saxatilis*. California Fish Game, 60(3): 128–131.

Korte F (1969) Summary of results in 1969. Unpublished report, submitted to WHO by Shell.

Korte F, Klein W, Weisgerber I, Kaul R, Mueller W, & Djirsurai A (1970) Recent results in studies on the fate of chlorinated insecticides. In: Deichmann WB, Radomski JL, & Penalver RA, ed. Proceedings of the Sixth Conference on Toxicology and Occupational Medicine, Pesticide Symposia. Miami, Florida, Halos & Associates, Inc., pp 51–56.

Krantz WC, Mulhern BM, Bagley GE, Sprunt A, Ligas FJ, & Robertson WC Jr (1970) Organochlorine and heavy metal residues in bald eagle eggs. Pestic Monit J, 4(3): 136–140.

Kreitzer JF (1980) Effects of toxaphene and endrin at very low dietary concentrations on discrimination acquisition and reversal in bobwhite quail *Colinus virginianus*. Environ Pollut (Ser A), 23: 217–230.

Kreitzer JF & Heinz GH (1974) The effect of sub-lethal dosages of five pesticides and a polychlorinated biphenyl on the avoidance response of Coturnix quail chicks. Environ Pollut, 6: 21–29.

Kubiak TJ, Harris HJ, Smith LM, Schwartz TR, Stalling DL, Trick JA, Sileo L, Docjerty DE, & Erdman TC (1989) Microcontaminants and reproductive impairment of the Forster's tern on Green Bay, Lake Michigan—1983. Arch Environ Contam Toxicol, 18: 706–727.

Kudesia VP & Bali NP (1985) A study of pesticides in Kalinadi River and evaluation of toxicity of some pesticides on fish *Clarias batrachus*. Acta Cienc Indica, 10C(4): 245–254.

Kummer R & Van Sittert NJ (1984) Field study on health effects in farmers applying an endrin/DDT/MEP formulation by hand-held ULV to cotton in Ivory Coast. Unpublished report, The Hague, Shell Internationale Petroleum Maatschappij, submitted to WHO by Shell.

Kummer R & Van Sittert NJ (1986) Field studies on health effects from the application of two organophosphorus insecticide formulations by hand-held ULV to cotton. Toxicol Lett, 33: 7–24.

Kurata M, Hirose K, & Umeda M (1982) Inhibition of metabolic cooperation in Chinese hamster cells by organochlorine pesticides. Gann, **73**: 217–221.

Kurhekar MP, D'Souza FC, & Meghal SK (1975) Rapid method for extracting aldrin, dieldrin, and endrin from visceral material. J Assoc Off Anal Chem, **58**(3): 548–550.

Kutz FW, Yobs AR, & Yang HSC (1976) National pesticide monitoring programs. In: Lee RE Jr, ed. Air pollution from pesticides and agricultural processes. Cleveland, Ohio, CRC Press, pp 95–136.

Kutz F, Strassman S, & Yobs AR (1979a) Survey of pesticide residues and their metabolites in the general population of the United States. In: Berlin A, Wolff AH, & Hasegawa Y ed. Use of biological specimens to assess human exposure to environmental pollutants, The Hague, Martinus Nijhoff, pp 267–274.

Kutz FW, Strassman SC, & Sperling JF (1979b) Survey of selected organochlorine pesticides in the general population of the United States. Fiscal years 1970-1975. Ann NY Acad Sci, **320**: 60–68.

Lara WH & Barreto HHC (1972) [Chlorinated pesticide residues in water.] Rev Inst Adolfo Lutz, **32**: 69–74 (in Portuguese with English summary).

Lauer GJ, Nicholson HP, Cox WS, & Teasley JI (1966) Pesticide contamination of surface waters by sugar cane farming in Louisiana. Trans Am Fish Soc, **95**(3): 310–316.

Lawrence CH, Coleman RL, & Sowell WL (1968) Endrin induced trace metal alterations following acute exposure. Bull Environ Contam Toxicol, **3**(4): 229–239.

Leard RL, Grantham BJ, & Pessoney GF (1980) Use of selected freshwater bivalves for monitoring organochlorine pesticide residues in major Mississippi stream systems, 1972-73. Pestic Monit J, **14**(2): 47–52.

Lebel GL & Williams DT (1986) Determination of halogenated contaminants in human adipose tissue. J Assoc Off Anal Chem, **69**(3): 451–458.

Lichtenberg JJ, Eichelberger JW, Dressman RC, & Longbottom JE (1970) Pesticides in surface waters of the United States; a 5-year summary, 1964-1968. Pestic Monit J, **4**(2): 71–86.

Lopez-Avila V, Schoen S, Milanes J, & Beckert WF (1988) Single-laboratory evaluation of EPA method 8080 for determination of chlorinated pesticides and polychlorinated biphenyls in hazardous wastes. J Assoc Off Anal Chem, **71**(2): 375–387.

Lowe JI (1966) Some effects of endrin on estuarine fishes. In: Proceedings of the 19th Annual Conference of the Southeast Association of Game and Fish Commissioners, pp 271–276.

References

Luckens MM & Davis WH (1965) Toxicity of dieldrin and endrin to bats. Nature, **207**(4999): 879–880.

Luckens MM & Phelps KI (1969) Serum enzyme patterns in acute poisoning with organochlorine insecticides. J Pharm Sci, **58**(5): 569–572.

Ludke JL (1976) Organochlorine pesticide residues associated with mortality: additivity of chlordane and endrin. Bull Environ Contam Toxicol, **16**(3): 253–260.

Luke MA, Masumoto HT, Cairns T, & Hundley HK (1988) Levels and incidences of pesticide residues in various foods and animal feeds analyzed by the Luke multi-residue methodology for fiscal years 1982-1986. J Assoc Off Anal Chem, **71**(2): 415–433.

Lund AE & Narahasi T (1983) Kinetics of sodium channel modification as the basis for the variation in the nerve membrane effects of pyrethroids and DDT analogs. Pestic Biochem Physiol, **20**: 203–206.

Lykins BW Jr, Koffskey WE, & Miller RG (1986) Chemical products and toxicologic effects of disinfection. J Am Water Works Assoc, **78**(11): 66–75.

McFall JA, Antoine SR, & Deleon IR (1985) Organics in the water column of Lake Pontchartrain. Chemosphere, **14**(9): 1253–1265.

McGill AEJ & Robinson J (1968) Organochlorine insecticide residues in complete prepared meals: a 12-month survey in SE England. Food Cosmet Toxicol, **6**: 45–57.

Machbub B, Ludwig HF, & Gunaratnam D (1988) Environmental impact from agrochemicals in Bali (Indonesia). Environ Monit Assess, **11**: 1–23.

McIntyre AE & Lester JN (1984) Occurrence and distribution of persistent organochlorine compounds in UK sewage sludges. Water Air Soil Pollut, **23**: 397–415.

McKenney CL Jr (1986) Critical responses of populations of crustacea to toxicants. Gulf Breeze, Florida, US Environmental Protection Agency, Environmental Research Laboratory (Environmental Research Brief EPA/600/M-86/004.

McLeese DW & Metcalfe CD (1980) Toxicities of eight organochlorine compounds in sediment and seawater to *Crangon septemspinosa*. Bull Environ Contam Toxicol **25**: 921-928.

McLeese DW, Metcalfe CD, & Pezzack DS (1980) Bioaccumulation of chlorobiphenyls and endrin from food by lobsters (*Homarus americanus*). Bull Environ Contam Toxicol **25**: 161-168.

McLeese DW, Burridge LE, & van Dinter J (1982) Toxicities of five organochlorine compounds in water and sediment to *Nereis virens*. Bull Environ Contam Toxicol **28**: 216-220.

Madden JD, Finerty MW, & Grodner RM (1989) Survey of persistent pesticide residues in the edible tissues of wild and pond-raised Louisiana crayfish and their habitat. Bull Environ Contam Toxicol, **43**: 779–784.

Manske DD & Corneliussen PE (1974) Pesticide residues in total diet samples (VII). Pestic Monit J, **8**(2): 110–124.

Manske DD & Johnson RD (1975) Pesticide residues in total diet samples (VIII). Pestic Monit J, **9**(2): 94–105.

Manske DD & Johnson RD (1977) Pesticide and other chemical residues in total diet samples (X). Pestic Monit J, **10**(4): 134–148.

Marinelli P, Stracciari GL, & Anfossi P (1986) [Presence of organochlorinated pesticides in some wine-making by-products.] Zoot Nutr Anim, **12**: 479–486 (in Italian with English summary).

Marsh C (1963) Metabolism of D-glucuronolactone in mammalian systems. Conversion of D-glucuronolactone into D-glucaric acid by tissue preparations. Biochem J, **87**: 82–90.

Marston RB, Tyo RM, & Middendorff SC (1969) Endrin in water from treated Douglas fir seed. Pestic Monit J, **2**(4): 167–171.

Martin RJ & Duggan RE (1968) Pesticide residues in total diet samples (III). Pestic Monit J, **1**(4): 11–20.

Martin DB & Hartman WA (1985) Organochlorine pesticides and polychlorinated biphenyls in sediment and fish from wetlands in the North Central United States. J Assoc Off Anal Chem, **68**(4): 712–717.

Martin JP, Harding RB, Cannell GH, & Anderson L (1959) Influence of five annual field applications of organic insecticides on soil biological and physical properties. Soil Sci, **87**: 334–338.

Maslansky CJ & Williams GM (1981) Evidence for an epigenetic mode of action in organochlorine pesticide hepatocarcinogenicity. A lack of genotoxicity in rat, mouse and hamster hepatocytes. J Toxicol Environ Health, **8**: 121–130.

Mason JW & Rowe OR (1976) The accumulation and loss of dieldrin and endrin in the eastern oyster. Arch Environ Contam Toxicol, **4**(3): 349–360.

Masud SZ & Farhat S (1985) Pesticide residues in foodstuffs in Pakistan—organochlorine pesticides in fruits and vegetables. Pak J Sci Ind Res, **28**(6): 417–422.

Matsumoto K, Eldefrawi ME, & Eldefrawi AT (1988) Action of polychlorocycloalkane insecticides on binding of [35S]t-butylbicyclophosphorothionate to *Torpedo* electric organ membranes and stereospecificity of binding site. Toxicol Appl Pharmacol, **95**: 220–229.

References

Matsumura F, Khanvilkar VG, Patil KC, & Boush GM (1971) Metabolism of endrin by certain soil microorganisms. J Agric Food Chem, **19**(1): 27–31.

Maule A, Plyte S, & Quirk AV (1987) Dehalogenation of organochlorine insecticides by mixed anaerobic microbial populations. Pestic Biochem Physiol, **27**: 229–236.

Mayer, FL Jr (1987) Acute toxicity handbook of chemicals to estuarine organisms. Gulf Breeze, Florida, US Environmental Protection Agency, Environmental Research Laboratory (Environmental Research Brief EPA/600/8-87/017).

Mayer FL Jr & Ellersieck MR (1986) Manual of acute toxicity: Interpretation and data base for 410 chemicals and 66 species of freshwater animals. Washington, DC, US Department of the Interior Fish and Wildlife Service (Resource publication 160).

Meena K, Gupta PK, & Bawa SR (1978) Endrin-induced toxicity in normal and irradiated rats. Environ Res, **16**: 373–382.

Mehrotra BD, Moorthy, KS, Reddy SR, & Desaiah D (1989) Effects of cyclodiene compounds on calcium pump activity in rat brain and heart. Toxicology, **54**: 17–29.

Meith-Avcin N, Warlen SM, & Barber RT (1973) Organochlorine insecticide residues in a bathyl-demersal fish from 2500 meters. Environ Lett, **5**(4): 215–221.

Mersch-Sundermann V, Dickgiesser N, Hablizel U, & Gruber B (1988) [Examination of mutagenicity of organic microcontaminations on the environment. I. Communication: the mutagenicity of selected herbicides and insecticides with the *Salmonella*-microsome-test (Ames-test) in consideration of the pathogenetic potence of contaminated ground- and drinking-water.] Zbl Bakteriol Hyg B, **186**: 247–260 (in German).

Metcalf RL, Kapoor IP, Lu PY, Schuth CK, & Sherman P (1973) Model ecosystem studies of the environmental fate of six organochlorine pesticides. Environ Health Perspect, **4**: 35–44.

Miles JRW & Harris CR (1973) Organochlorine insecticides residues in streams draining agricultural, urban agricultural and resort areas of Ontario, Canada, 1971. Pestic Monit J, **6**(4): 363–368.

Miller PE & Fink GB (1973) Brain serotonin level and pentylenetetrazol seizure threshold in dieldrin and endrin treated mice. Proc West Pharmacol Soc, **16**: 195–197.

Modin JC (1969) Chlorinated hydrocarbon pesticides in California bays and estuaries. Pestic Monit J, **3**(1): 1–7.

Morita H & Umeda M (1984) Detection of mutagenicity of various compounds by FM3A cell system. Mutat Res, **130**(5): 371.

Moriya M, Ohta T, Watanabe K, Miyazawa T, Kato K, & Shirasu Y (1983) Further mutagenicity studies on pesticides in bacterial reversion assay system. Mutat Res, **116**: 185–216.

Morris RD (1968) Effects of endrin feeding on survival and reproduction in the deer mouse, *Peromyscus maniculatus*. Can J Zool, **46**(5): 951–958.

Morris RD (1970) The effects of endrin on *Microtus* and *Peromyscus*. I. Unenclosed field populations. Can J Zool, **48**: 695–708.

Morris RD (1972) The effects of endrin on *Microtus* and *Peromyscus*. II. Enclosed field populations. Can J Zool, **50**(6): 885–896.

Moser GJ & Smart RC (1989) Hepatic tumour-promoting chlorinated hydrocarbons stimulate protein kinase C activity. Carcinogenesis, **10**(5): 851–856.

Mount DI & Putnicki GJ (1966) Summary report of the 1963 Mississippi fish kill. North Am Wildl Nat Res Conf Trans, **31**: 177–184.

Mount DI, Vigor LW, & Schafer ML (1966) Endrin: use of concentration in blood to diagnose acute toxicity in fish. Science, **152**: 1388–1390.

Mugambi JM, Kanja L, Maitho TE, Skaare JU, & Lokken P (1989) Organochlorine pesticide residues in domestic fowl (*Gallus domesticus*) eggs from Central Kenya. J Sci Food Agric, **48**: 165–176.

Muir CMC (1970) The acute oral and percutaneous toxicities to rats of formulations of aldrin, dieldrin or endrin. Unpublished report No. TLGR.0020.70, Sittingbourne, Kent, Shell Research, submitted to WHO by Shell.

Mukerjee SK (1985) The environmental photodegradation of pesticides. Indian J Agric Chem, **18**(1): 1–9.

Mulhern BM, Reichel WL, Locke LN, Lamont TG, Belisle A, Cromartie E, Bagerly GE, & Prouty R (1970) Organochlorine residues and autopsy data from bald eagles. 1966-1968. Pestic Monit J, **4**: 141–144.

Muncy RJ & Oliver AD Jr (1963) Toxicity of ten insecticides to the red crawfish, *Procambarus clarki* (Girard). Trans Am Fish Soc, **92**: 428–431.

Mussalo-Rauhamaa H, Salmela SS, Leppanen A, & Pyysalo H (1986) Cigarettes as a source of some trace and heavy metals and pesticides in man. Arch Environ Health, **41**(1): 49–55.

References

Nagelsmit A, Vliet PW, van Wiel-Wetzels WAM, van der Wielard MJ, Strik JJTWA, Ottevanger CF, & van Sittert NJ (1979) Porphyrins as possible parameters for exposure to hexachlorocyclopentadiene, allylchloride, epichlorohydrin and endrin. In: Strik JJTWA & Koeman JH, ed. Chemical porphyria in man. Amsterdam, Elsevier/North Holland Biochemical Press, pp 55–61.

Narahasi T (1987) Effects of toxic agents on neural membranes. In: Lowndes HE, ed. Electrophysiology in neurotoxicology. Boca Raton, Florida, CRC Press, vol 1, pp 23–44.

NCI (1978) Bioassay of endrin for possible carcinogenicity. Bethesda, Maryland, Department of Health Education, and Welfare, National Cancer Institute (DHEW Publication No. NIH 179-812)

NCI (1979) Bioassay of endrin for possible carcinogenicity. Bethesda, Maryland, Department of Health Education, and Welfare, National Cancer Institute, 110 pp (Carcinogenesis Technical Report Series No. 12; NTIS PB-288461)

Nebeker AV, Schuytema GS, Griffis WL, Barbitta JA, & Carey LA (1989) Effect of sediment organic carbon on survival of Hyalella azteca exposed to DDT and endrin. Environ Toxicol Chem, **8**: 705–718.

Nelson SC, Bahler TL, Hartwell WV, Greenwood DA, & Harris LE (1956) Serum alkaline phosphatase levels, weight changes and mortality rates of rats fed endrin. J Agric Food Chem, **4**(8): 696–700.

Nettleship DN & Peakall DB (1987) Organochlorine residue levels in three high Arctic species of colonially-breeding seabirds from Prince Leopold Island. Mar Pollut Bull, **18**(8): 434–438.

NIOSH (1989) Manual of analytical methods. Endrin: Method No. 5519. Cincinnati, Ohio, National Institute for Occupational Safety and Health, pp 1–4.

Nishimura N, Nishimura H, & Oshima H (1982) Survey on mutagenicity of pesticides by the Salmonella-microsome test. J Aichi Med Univ Assoc, **10**(4): 305–312.

Notten WRF & Henderson PT (1975) Alteration in urinary D-glucaric acid excretion as an indication of exposition to xenobiotics. In: Proceedings of the International Symposium—Environment and Health, CEC/EPA/WHO, Paris, 1974.

Novak AF & Rao MRR (1965) Food safety program: endrin monitoring in the Mississippi River. Science, **150**: 1751.

Ohlendorf HM, Swineford DM, & Locke LN (1981) Organochlorine residues and mortality of herons. Pestic Monit J, **14**(4): 125–135.

Onodera S & Tabucanon MS (1986) Organochlorine pesticide residues in the lower Chao Phraya River and klongs along the river at Bangkok metropolitan area, 1982-1984. J Sci Soc Thailand, **12**: 225–238.

Oomen PA (1986) A sequential scheme for evaluating the hazard of pesticides to bees, *Apis mellifera*. Meded Fac Landbouwwet Rijksuniv Gent, **51**(3b): 1205–1213.

Osborne BG, Barrett GM, Laal-Khoshab A, & Willis K (1989) The occurrence of pesticide residues in UK home-grown and imported wheat. Pestic Sci, **27**: 103–109.

O'Shea TJ, Brownell RL Jr, Clarke DR Jr, Walker WA, Gay ML, & Lamont TG (1980) Organochlorine pollutants in small cetaceans from the Pacific and South Atlantic Oceans, November 1968-June 1976. Pestic Monit J, **14**:(2): 35–46.

Ottevanger CF & Van Sittert NJ (1979) Relation between anti-12-hydroxy endrin excretion and enzyme induction in workers involved in the manufacture of endrin. In: Strik JJTWA & Koeman JH, ed. Chemical porphyria in man. Amsterdam, Elsevier/North Holland Biomedical Press, pp 123–129.

Ottolenghi AD, Haseman JK, & Suggs F (1974) Teratogenic effects of aldrin, dieldrin and endrin in hamsters and mice. Teratology, **9**: 11–16.

Parveen Z & Masud SZ (1987) Organochlorine pesticide residues in cattle feed samples in Karachi, Pakistan. J Sci Ind Res; **30**(7): 513–516.

Patil KC, Matsumura F, & Boush GM (1970) Degradation of endrin, aldrin, and DDT by soil microorganisms. Appl Microbiol, **19**(5): 879–881.

Pavan I, Buglione E, Pettinati L, Perrelli G, Rubino GF, Bicchi C, D'Amato A, Carlino F, Bugiani M, & Polizzi S (1987) [Accumulation of organochlorine pesticides in human adipose tissue. data from the province of Turin (Italy).] Med Lav, **78**(3): 219–228 (in Italian).

Pawar SS & Kachole MS (1978) Hepatic and renal microsomal electron transport reactions in endrin treated female guinea pigs. Bull Environ Contam Toxicol, **20**: 199–205.

Pearce F (1987) Pesticide deaths: the price of the green revolution. New Sci, **114**: 30.

Peterson SR & Ellarson RS (1978) pp'-DDE, polychlorinated biphenyls, and endrin in old squaws in North America, 1969-73. Pestic Monit J, **11**(4): 170–181.

Petrella VJ, Fox JP, & Webb RE (1975) Endrin metabolism in endrin-susceptible and resistant strains of pine mice. Toxicol Appl Pharmacol, **34**: 283–291.

Petrella VJ, McKinney JD, Fox JP, & Webb RE (1977) Identification of metabolites of endrin. Metabolism in endrin susceptible and resistant strains of pine mice. J Agric Food Chem, **25**(2): 393–398.

Pfister RM (1972) Interactions of halogenated pesticides and microorganisms: a review. CRC Crit Rev Microbiol, **21**(1): 1–33.

Phillips DD, Pollard GE, & Soloway SB (1962) Thermal isomerization of endrin and its behaviour in gas chromatography. J Agric Food Chem, **10**(3): 217–221.

References

Plimmer JR (1972) Photochemistry of organochlorine insecticides. In: Tahori AS, ed. Proceedings of the Ssecond international IUPAC congress of pesticides chemistry. New York, Gordon & Breach, vol 1, pp 413–432.

Podrebarac DS (1984) Pesticide, heavy metal, and other chemical residues in infant and toddler total diet samples (IV). October 1977–September 1978. J Assoc Off Anal Chem, **67**(1): 166–175.

Probst GS, McMahon RE, Hill LE, Thompson CZ, Epp JK, & Neal SB (1981) Chemically-induced unscheduled DNA synthesis in primary rat hepatocyte cultures: a comparison with bacterial mutagenicity using 218 compounds. Environ Mutagen, **3**: 11–32.

Prouty RM & Bunck C (1986) Organochlorine residues in adult mallard and black duck wings, 1981-1982. Environ Monit Assess, **6**: 49–57.

Prouty RM, Reichel WL, Locke LN, Belisle AA, Cromartie E, Kaiser TE, Lamont TG, Mulhern BM, & Swineford DM (1977) Residues of organochlorine pesticides and polychlorinated biphenyls and autopsy data for bald eagles, 1973–74. Pestic Monit J, **11**: 134–137.

Radeleff RD (1956) Hazards to livestock of insecticides used in mosquito control. Mosq News, **16**(2): 79–80.

Radhakrishnan AG & Antony PD (1989) Pesticide residues in marine fishes. Fish Technol, **26**: 60–61.

Rashid KA & Mumma RO (1986) Screening pesticides for their ability to damage bacterial DNA. J Environ Sci Health, **B21**(4): 319–334.

Reddy DB, Edward VD, Abraham GJS, & Rao KV (1966) Fatal endrin poisoning. A detailed autopsy, histopathological and experimental study. J Indian Med Assoc, **46**(3): 121–124.

Reddy DB, Abraham GJS, Edward VD, Naganna B, & Mathalli M (1967) Further observations on endrin poisoning. J Indian Med Prof, **13**(10): 5946, 5967–5968.

Redetzke K., Gonzalez AA, & Applegate HG (1983) Organochlorine pesticides in adipose tissue of persons from Ciudad Juarez, Mexico. J Environ Health, **46**(1): 25–27.

Reece RL, Scott PC, Forsyth WM, Gould JA, & Barr DA (1985) Toxicity episodes involving agricultural chemicals and other substances in birds in Victoria, Australia. Vet Rec, **117**(20): 525–527.

Reeves RG, Woodham DW, Ganyard MC, & Bond CA (1977) Preliminary monitoring of agricultural pesticides in a cooperative tobacco pest management project in North Carolina, 1971—first-year study. Pestic Monit J, **11**(2): 99–106.

Reichel WL, Lamont TG, Cromartie E, & Locke LN (1969) Residues in two bald eagles suspected of pesticide poisoning. Bull Environ Contam Toxicol, 4(1): 24–30.

Reidinger RF & Crabtree DG (1974) Organochlorine residues in golden eagles, United States—March 1964-July 1971. Pestic Monit J, 8(1): 37–43.

Reins DA, Holmes DD, & Hinshaw LB (1964) Acute and chronic effects of the insecticide endrin on renal function and renal hemodynamics. Can J Physiol Pharmacol, 42(5): 599–608.

Reins DA, Rieger JA Jr, Stavinoha WB, & Hinshaw LB (1966) Effect of endrin on venous return and catecholamine release in the dog. Can J Physiol Pharmacol, 44: 59–67.

Ressang AA, Titus I, Andar RS, & Soedarmo D (1958) Aldrin, dieldrin and endrin intoxication in cats. Commun Vet, 2(2): 71–88.

Reuber MD (1978) Carcinomas, sarcomas and other lesions in Osborne-Mendel rats ingesting endrin. Exp Cell Biol, 46(3): 129–145.

Revzin AM (1966) Effects of endrin on telencephalic function in the pigeon. Toxicol Appl Pharmacol, 9(1): 75–83.

Revzin AM (1980) Some acute and chronic effects of endrin on the brains of pigeons and monkeys. In: Proceedings of the symposium on the biological impact of pesticides in the environment, pp 134–141.

Ribbens PH (1985) Mortality study of industrial workers exposed to aldrin, dieldrin and endrin. Arch Occup Environ Health, 56(2): 75–79.

Richardson LA, Lane JR, Gardner WS, Peeler JT, & Campbell JE (1967) Relationship of dietary intake to concentration of dieldrin and endrin in dogs. Bull Environ Contam Toxicol, 2(4): 207–219.

Richardson A, Robinson J, & Baldwin MK (1970) Metabolism of endrin in the rat. Chem Ind, 1970,: 502–503.

Ritchey SJ, Young RW, & Essary EO (1972) Effects of heating and cooking method on chlorinated hydrocarbon residues in chicken tissues. J Agric Food Chem, 20: 291–293.

Robinson J & McGill AEJ (1966) Organochlorine insecticide residues in complete prepared meals in Great Britain during 1965. Nature, 212(5066): 1037–1038.

Robinson J, Richardson A, Hunter CG, Crabtree AN, & Rees HJ (1965) Organochlorine insecticide content of human adipose tissue in south-eastern England. Br J Ind Med, 22: 220–229.

References

Roos AH, van Munsteren AJ, Nab FM, & Tuinstra LGMT (1987) Universal extraction/clean-up procedure for screening of pesticides by extraction with ethylacetate and size exclusion chromatography. Anal Chim Acta, **196**: 95–102.

Rosales MTL, Escalona RL, Alarcon RM, & Zamora V (1985) Organochlorine hydrocarbon residues in sediments of two different lagoons of Northwest Mexico. Bull Environ Contam Toxicol, **35**: 322–330.

Rosen JD (1972) Conversion of pesticides under environmental conditions. In: Coulston F & Korte F ed. Environmental quality. Stuttgart, George Thieme, vol 1, pp 85–96.

Rosen JD, Sutherland DJ, & Lipton GR (1966) The photochemical isomerization of dieldrin and endrin and effects on toxicity. Bull Environ Contam Toxicol, **1**: 133–140.

Rowe DR, Canter LW, Snyder PJ, & Mason JW (1971) Dieldrin and endrin concentrations in a Louisiana estuary. Pestic Monit J, **4**(4): 177–183.

Rowley DL, Rab MA, Hardjotanojo W, Liddle J, Burse VW, Saleem M, Sokal D, Falk H, & Head SL (1987) Convulsions caused by endrin poisoning in Pakistan. Pediatrics, **79**(6): 928–934.

Roylance KJ, Jorgensen CD, Booth GM, & Carter MW (1985) Effects of dietary endrin on reproduction of Mallard ducks (*Anas platyrhynchos*). Arch Environ Contam Toxicol, **14**: 705–711.

Runhaar EA, Sangster B, Greve PA, & Voortman M (1985) A case of fatal endrin poisoning. Hum Toxicol, **4**: 241–247.

Ryan S, Bacher GJ, & Martin AA (1972) The mussel *Hyridella australis* as a biological monitor of the pesticide endrin in fresh water. Search, 3(11–12): 446–447.

Safe S & Hutzinger O (1979) Mass spectrometry of pesticides and pollutants. Boca Raton, Florida, CRC Press, Inc.

Saiki MK & Schmitt CJ (1986) Organochlorine chemical residues in bluegills and common carp from the irrigated San Joaquin Valley floor, California. Arch Environ Contam Toxicol, **15**: 357–366.

Samhan O & Ghobrial F (1987) Trace metals and chlorinated hydrocarbons in sewage sludges of Kuwait. Water Air Soil Pollut, **36**: 239–246.

Satsmadjis J, Georgakopoulos-Gregoriades E, & Voutsinou-Taliadouri F (1988) Red mullet contamination by PCBs and chlorinated pesticides in the Pagassitikos Gulf, Greece. Mar Pollut Bull, **19**(3): 136–138.

Schafer ML, Peeler JT, Gardner WS, & Campbell JE (1969) Pesticides in drinking water—waters from the Mississippi and Missouri rivers. Environ Sci Technol, 3(12): 1261–1269.

Schafer EW Jr, Bowles WA Jr, & Hurlbut J (1983) The acute oral toxicity, repellency, and hazard potential of 998 chemicals to one or more species of wild and domestic birds. Arch Environ Contam Toxicol, 12: 355–382.

Scheutz EG, Wrighton SA, Safe SH, & Guzelian PS (1986) Regulation of cytochrome P-450p by phenobarbital and phenobarbital-like inducers in adult rat hepatocytes in primary monolayer culture and in vivo. Biochemistry, 25: 1124–1133.

Schwabe U & Wendling I (1967) [Stimulation of drug metabolism by low doses of DDT and other chlorinated hydrocarbon insecticides.] Arzneimittel-forschung, 17(5): 614–618 (in German).

Seifert J (1988) Ontogenesis and properties of the convulsant recognition site(s) of the gamma-aminobutyric acid (GABA) receptor complex in chicken embryo. Eur J Pharmacol, 151: 443–448.

Seifert J (1989) Teratogenesis of polychlorocycloalkane insecticides in chicken embryos resulting from their interactions at the convulsant recognition sites of the GABA (pro)receptor complex. Bull Environ Contam Toxicol, 42: 707–715.

Sherman M & Rosenberg M (1954) Subchronic toxicity of four chlorinated dimethanonaphthalene insecticides to chicks. J Econ Entomol, 47(6): 1082–1083.

Sierra M & Santiago D (1987) Organochlorine pesticide levels in barn owls collected in Leon, Spain. Bull Environ Contam Toxicol, 38: 261–265.

Sierra M, Teran MT, Gallego A, Diez MJ, & Santiago D (1987) Organochlorine contamination in three species of diurnal raptors in Leon, Spain. Bull Environ Contam Toxicol, 38: 254–260.

Simmon VF, Kauhanen K, & Tardiff RC (1977) Mutagenic activity of chemicals identified in drinking water. In: Scott D, Bridges BA, & Sobels FH ed. Progress in genetic toxicology. Amsterdam, Elsevier/North Holland Biomedical Press, pp 249–258.

Singh MN (1988) Mortality response of *Achatina fulica* to various pesticides. J Environ Biol, 9(2): 157–162.

Singh PDA & West ME (1985) Acute pesticide poisoning in the Caribbean. West Indian Med J, 34: 75–83.

Singhal RL & Kacew S (1976) The role of cyclic AMP in chlorinated hydrocarbon-induced toxicity. Fed Proc, 35(14): 2618–2623.

Smith KJ, Polen PB, de Vries DM, & Coon FB (1968) Removal of chlorinated pesticides from crude vegetable oils by simulated commercial processing procedures. J Am Oil Chem Soc, 45: 866–869.

References

Sobti RC, Krishan A, & Davies J (1983) Cytokinetic and cytogenetic effect of agricultural chemicals on human lymphoid cells *in vitro*. II. Organochlorine pesticides. Arch Toxicol, **52**: 221–231.

Somers JD, Goski BC, & Barrett MW (1987) Organochlorine residues in northeastern Alberta otters. Bull Environ Contam Toxicol, **39**: 783–790.

Soto AR & Deichmann WB (1967) Major metabolism and acute toxicity of aldrin, dieldrin and endrin. Environ Res, **1**(4): 307–322.

Spann JW, Heinz GH, & Hulse CS (1986) Reproduction and health of mallards fed endrin. Environ Toxicol Chem, **5**: 755–759.

Speck LB & Maaske CA (1958) The effects of chronic and acute exposure of rats to endrin. Arch Ind Health, **18**: 268–272.

Spynu EI (1964) On the toxicology of new organic chloride insecticides obtained by diene synthesis on the basis of hexachlorocyclopentadiene. Gig Tr Prof Zabol, **4**: 30–35.

Squires RF & Saederup E (1989) Polychlorinated convulsant insecticides potentiate the protective effect of NaCl against heat inactivation of [3H] fluonitrazepam binding sites. J Neurochem, **52**: 537–543.

Stanford Research Institute (1953) Unpublished letter Report No. 1 Ref. Project No. B-868 November 10, Stanford, CA, submitted to WHO by Shell.

Stanford Research Institute (1954) Unpublished letter Report No. 3 Ref. Project No. B-868 February 1, Stanford, CA, submitted to WHO by Shell.

Stanley CW, Barney JE II, Helton MR, & Yobs AR (1971) Measurement of atmospheric levels of pesticides. Environ Sci Technol, **5**: 430–435.

Steinberg KK, Garza A, Bueso JA, Burse VW, & Phillips DL (1989) Serum pesticide concentrations in farming cooperatives in Honduras. Bull Environ Contam Toxicol, **42**: 643–650.

Stickel WH, Kaiser TE, & Reichel WL (1979) Endrin versus 12-ketoendrin in birds and rodents. In: Kenaga EE ed. Avian and mammalian wildlife toxicology, Philadeplphia,, American Society for Testing and Materials, pp 61–68 (ASTM STP 693).

Stout VF (1980) Organochlorine residues in fishes from the Northwest Atlantic Ocean and Gulf of Mexico. Fish Bull, **78**(1): 51–58.

Strachan WMJ (1988) Toxic contaminants in rainfall in Canada: 1984. Environ Toxicol Chem, **7**: 871–877.

Strachan WMJ, Huneault H, Schertzer WM, & Elder FC (1980) Organochlorines in precipitation in the Great Lakes region. In: Afghan BK & MacKay D ed. Hydrocarbons and halogenated hydrocarbons in the aquatic environment. New York, Plenum Publishing Corp., pp 387–396.

Strassman SC & Kutz FW (1977) Insecticide residues in human milk from Arkansas and Mississippi, 1973–1974. Pestic Monit J, 10(4): 130–133.

Strik JJTWA (1979) The occurrence of chronic hepatic porphyria in man, caused by halogenated hydrocarbons. In: Strik JJTWA & Koeman JH ed. Chemical porphyria in man. Amsterdam, Elsevier/North Holland Biomedical Press, p 3.

Struger J, Weseloh D, Hallett DJ, & Mineau P (1985) Organochlorine contaminants in herring gull eggs from the Detroit and Niagara Rivers and Saginaw Bay (1978-1982): contaminant discriminants. J Great Lakes Res, 11(3): 223–230.

Sturm R, Knauth HD, Reinhardt KH, & Gandrasz J (1986) Distribution of chlorinated hydrocarbons in sediment and seston of the River Elbe. Wasser, 67: 23–38.

Sundershan P & Khan MAQ (1980) Metabolic fate of [^{14}C] endrin in bluegill fish. Pestic Biochem Physiol, 14: 5–12.

Suzuki M & Morimoto M (986) High resolution chemically bonded fused-silica capillary gas chromatography of organochlorine insecticides and related compounds in arable soil samples. J High Resol Chromatogr Chromatogr Commun, 9: 296–298.

Suzuki M, Yamato Y, & Watanabe T (1973) Multiple organochlorine pesticide residues in Japan. Bull Environ Contam Toxicol, 10(3): 145–150.

Suzuki K, Nagayoshi H, & Kashiwa T (1974) The systematic separation and identification of pesticide in the first division. Agric Biol Chem, 38(2): 279–285.

Sykes PW Jr (1985) Pesticide concentrations in snail kite eggs and nestlings in Florida. Condor, 87: 438.

Tarrant KR & Tatton JO'G (1968) Organochlorine pesticides in rainwater in the British Isles. Nature, 219(5155): 725–727.

Telling GM, Sissons DJ, & Brinkman HW (1977) Determination of organochlorine insecticide residues in fatty food stuffs using a clean-up technique based on a single column of activated alumina. J Chromatogr, 137: 405–423.

Teran MT & Sierra M (1987) Organochlorine insecticides in trout, *Salmo trutta fario* L. taken from four rivers in Leon, Spain. Bull Environ Contam Toxicol, 38: 247–253.

Terriere LC (1964) Endrin. In: Zweig, G ed. Analytical methods for pesticides, plant growth regulators and food additives. New York, Academic Press, vol 2, pp 209–222.

References

Terriere LC, Kiigemagi U, & England DC (1958) Endrin content of body tissues of steers, lambs and hogs receiving endrin in their daily diet. J Agric Food Chem, **6**(7): 516–518.

Terriere LC, Arscott GH, & Kiigemagi U (1959) The endrin content of eggs and body tissue of poultry receiving endrin in their daily diet. J Agric Food Chem, **7**(7): 502–504.

Thier HP & Stijve T (1986) [Results of an inter-laboratory comparison of analyses of analyses of organochlorine and organophosphorus pesticide residues in fat.] Lebensmittelchem Gerichtl Chem, **40**: 73–75 (in German).

Thompson JF (1976) Manual of analytical quality control for pesticides and related compounds in human and environmental samples. Research Triangle Park, North Carolina, US Environmental Protection Agency, Office of Research and Development, Health Effects Research Laboratory (EPA-600/1-76-017).

Thurston R, Gilfoil TA, Meyn EL, Zajdel RK, Aoki TI, & Veith GD (1985) Comparative toxicity of ten organic chemicals to ten common aquatic species. Water Res, **19**(9): 1145–1155.

Travis CC & Arms AD (1988) Bioconcentration of organics in beef, milk and vegetation. Environ Sci Technol, **22**: 271–274.

Treon JF, Cleveland FP, & Cappel J (1955) Toxicity of endrin for laboratory animals. J Agric Food Chem, **3**(10): 842–848.

Truhaut R, Do Phuoc H, & Phu Lich N (1974) Influence de l'administration de pesticides organo-halogénés et de polychloro-biphényles sur le métabolisme de la zoxazolamine chez le rat. CR Acad Sci Paris Sér D, **278**: 3003–3006.

Tucker RK & Crabtree DG (1970) Handbook of toxicity of pesticides to wildlife. Washington, DC, US Bureau of Sport Fisheries and Wildlife, Denver Wildlife Center (Resource Publication No. 84).

Tuinstra LGMT (1971) Organochlorine insecticide residues in human milk in the Leiden region. Neth Milk Dairy J, **25**: 24–32.

Uhnak J, Sackmauerova M, Szokolay A, & Pal'usova O (1974) The use of an electron capture detector for the determination of pesticides in water. J Chromatogr **91**: 545-547.

United Kingdom Ministry of Agriculture, Fisheries and Food (1989) Report of the Working Party on Pesticide Residues 1985–1988. London, Her Majesty's Stationery Office (Food Surveillance Paper No. 25).

US EPA (1974) New Orleans area water supply study (draft analytical report). Dallas, Texas, US Environmental Protection Agency, Lower Mississippi River Facility, Surveillance and Analysis Divisions, Region VI.

US EPA (1983) Findings of selected chemical residues in human blood serum and adipose tissue: Endrin. Environ News, **9 May**.

US EPA (1985) Hexachloronorbornadiene; Proposed submission of notice of manufacturer, import or processing and determination of significant new use. Fed Reg, **50**(36): 7351–7356.

US EPA (1987a) Health effects assessment for endrin. Cincinnati, Ohio, US Environmental Protection Agency, Ofice of Research and Development, Environmental Criteria and Assessment Office, 31 pp (Report PB88-180237).

US EPA (1987b) Health advisories for 16 pesticides. Washington, DC, US Environmental Protection Agency, Office of Drinking Water, 18 pp (Report PB87-200176).

Vance BD & Drummond W (1969) Biological concentration of pesticides by algae. J Am Water Works Assoc, **61**: 360–362.

Van Dijck P & van de Voorde H (1976) Mutagenicity versus carcinogenicity of organochlorine insecticides. Meded Fac Landbouww Rijksuniv Gent, **41**(2): 1491–1498.

Van Raalte HGS (1965) [Some aspects of pesticide toxicity.] Unpublished paper presented at the Conference on Occupational Health, Caracas, Venezuela; The Hague. Shell, International Petroleum Company, Health, Safety and Environment Division (in Spanish).

Van Sittert NJ (1985) Biological monitoring of bestrijdingsmiddelen; Coronel-PAOG Nascholingssymposium. Unpublished paper, Amsterdam, Vrije Universiteit, February 1985 (in Dutch).

Van Wynen JH & Stykel A (1988) Health risk assessment of residents living on harbour sludge. Arch Occup Environ Health, **61**: 77–87.

Veith GD, Kuehl DW, Leonard EN, Puglisi FA, & Lemke AE (1979) Polychlorinated biphenyls and other organic chemical residues in fish from major watersheds of the United States, 1976. Pestic Monit J, **13**(1): 1–11.

Veith GD, Kuehl DW, Leonard EN, Welch K, & Pratt G (1981) Polychlorinated biphenyls and other organic chemical residues in fish from major United States watersheds near the Great Lakes, 1978. Pestic Monit J, **15**(1): 1–8.

Verma MP, Bahga HS, Soni BK, & Singh SP (1970) Effect of insecticides on lactic acid concentration in the blood of buffalo-calves. Indian Vet J, **47**(12): 1056–1058.

Vermeer K, Risebrough RW, Spaans AL, & Reynolds LM (1974) Pesticide effects on fishes and birds in rice fields in Surinam, South America. Environ Pollut, **7**: 217–236.

Versteeg JPJ & Jager KW (1973) Long-term occupational exposure to the insecticides aldrin, dieldrin, endrin and telodrin. Br J Ind Med, **30**: 201–202.

References

Villeneuve JP, Holm E, & Cattini C (1985) Transfer of chlorinated hydrocarbons in the food chain lichen → reindeer → man. Chemosphere, **14**(11/12): 1651–1658.

Von Westernhagen H, Dethlefsen V, Cameron P, & Janssen D (1987) Chlorinated hydrocarbon residues in gonads of marine fish and effects on reproduction. Sarsia, **72**: 419–422.

Von Westernhagen H, Cameron P, Dethlefsen V, & Janssen D (1989) Chlorinated hydrocarbons in North Sea whiting (*Merlangius merlangus*) and effects on reproduction. I. Tissue burden and hatching success. Helgolander Meeresunters **43**: 45-60.

Vrij-Standhardt WG, Strik JJTWA, Ottevanger CF, & van Sittert NJ (1979) Urinary D-glucaric acid and urinary total porphyrin excretion in workers exposed to endrin. In: Strik JJTWA & Koeman JH ed. Chemical porphyria in man. Amsterdam, Elsevier/North Holland Biomedical Press, pp 113–121.

Wafford KA, Sattelle DB, Gant DB, Eldefrawi AT, & Eldefrawi ME (1989a) Non-competitive inhibition of GABA receptors in insect and vertebrate CNS by endrin and lindane. Pestic Biochem Physiol, **33**: 213–219.

Wafford KA, Lummis SCR, & Sattelle DB (1989b) Block of an insect central nervous system GABA receptor by cyclodiene and cyclohexane insecticides. Proc R Soc Lond, **B237**: 53–61.

Walker JJ & Phillips DE (1987) An electron microscopic study of endrin induced alterations in unmyelinated fibers of mouse sciatic nerve. Neurotoxicology, **8**(1): 55–64.

Walsh GM & Fink GB (1970) Temporal aspects of acute endrin toxicity in mice. Proc West Pharmacol Soc, **13**: 81–83.

Walsh GM & Fink GB (1972) Comparative toxicity and ditribution of endrin and dieldrin after intravenous administration in mice. Toxicol Appl Pharmacol, **23**: 408–416.

Wang HH & MacMahon B (1979) Mortality of workers employed in the manufacture of chlordane and heptachlor. J Occup Med, **21**(11):745–748.

Wassermann M, Curnow DH, Forte PN, & Groner Y (1968) Storage of organochlorine pesticides in the body fat of people in Western Australia. Int J Ind Med Surg, **37**(4): 295–300.

Wassermann M, Francone MP, Wassermann D, Mariani F, & Groner J (1969) [Organochlorine pesticide content of the fatty tissue of the general public in Argentina.] Sem Med, **134**(16): 459–462 (in Spanish).

Waters MD, Sandhu SS, Simmon VF, Mortelmans KE, Mitchell AD, Jorgenson TA, Jones DCL, Valencia R, & Garrett NE (1982) Study of pesticide genotoxicity. Basic Life Sci, **21**: 275–326.

Webb RE & Horsfall F Jr (1967) Endrin resistance in pine mouse. Science, **156**: 1762.

Webb RE, Hartgrove RW, Randolph WC, Petrella VJ, & Horsfall F Jr (1973) Toxicity studies in endrin-susceptible and resistant strains of pine mice. Toxicol Appl Pharmacol, **25**(1): 42–47.

Weeks DE (1967) Endrin food-poisoning. A report on four outbreaks caused by two separate shipments of endrin-contaminated flour. Bull World Health Organ, **37**: 499–512.

Wegman RCC & Greve PA (1974) Levels of organochlorine pesticides and inorganic bromide in human milk. Meded Fac Landbouwwet Rijksuniv Gent, **39**: 1301–1310.

Wegman RCC & Greve PA (1978) Organochlorines, cholinesterase inhibitors and aromatic amines in Dutch water samples, September 1969–December 1975. Pestic Monit J, **12**(3): 149–162.

Wegman RCC & Greve PA (1980) Halogenated hydrocarbons in Dutch water samples over the years 1969–1977. Environ Sci Res, **16**: 405–415.

Wegman RCC & Hofstee AWM (1982) Determination of organochlorines in river sediment by capillary gas chromatography. Water Res, **16**: 1265–1272.

Wegman RCC, Hofstee AWM, & Greve PA (1981) Uptake of organochlorines by plants growing on river and basin sediment. Meded Fac Landbouwwet Rijksuniv Gent, **46**(1): 359–365.

Weisgerber I, Klein W, & Korte F (1969) [Disappearance of residues and metabolism of endrin-(^{14}C) in tobacco.] Liebigs Ann Chem, **729**: 193–197 (in German with English abstract).

Wells MR & Yarbrough JD (1972) Vertebrate insecticide resistance: in vivo and in vitro endrin binding to cellular fractions from brain and liver tissues of Gambusia. J Agric Food Chem, **20**(1): 14–16.

Whetstone RR (1964) Chlorocarbons and chlorohydrocarbons: chlorinated derivatives of cyclopentadiene. In: Kirk-Othmer encyclopedia of chemical technology, 2nd ed., New York, John Wiley and Sons, vol 5, pp 240–252.

WHO (1989) Environmental Health Criteria No. 91: Aldrin and dieldrin. Geneva, World Health Organization, 335 pp.

WHO (1992) The WHO recommended classification of pesticides by hazard. Guidelines to classification 1992–1993. Geneva, World Health Organization (WHO/PCS/92.14).

WHO/FAO (1975) Data sheets on pesticides No. 1: Endrin. Geneva, World Health Organization (VBC/DS/75.1).

References

Wiemeyer SN, Jurek RM, & Moore JF (1986) Environmental contaminants in surrogates, foods and feathers of California condors (*Gymnogyps californianus*). Environ Monit Assess, **6**: 91–111.

Williams S (1964) Pesticide residues in total diet samples. J Assoc Off Anal Chem, **47**(5): 815–821.

Williams GM (1979) Liver cell culture systems for the study of hepatocarcinogenesis. In: Margison GP ed Advances in medical oncology research and education: Carcinogenesis, New York, Pergamon Press, vol 1, pp 273–280.

Williams S, Mills PA, & McDowell RE (1964) Residues in milk of cows fed rations containing low concentrations of five chlorinated hydrocarbon pesticides. J Asoc Off Agric Chem, **47**: 1124–1128.

Williams DT, Benoit FM, McNeil EE, & Otson R (1978) Organochlorine pesticide levels in Ottawa drinking water, 1976. Pestic Monit J, **12**(3): 163–166.

Williams DT, Lebel GL, & Junkins E (1984) A comparison of organochlorine residues in human adipose tissue autopsy samples from two Ontario municipalities. J Toxicol Environ Health, **13**: 19–29.

Williams DT, Lebel GL, & Junkins E (1988) Organohalogen residues in human adipose autopsy samples from six Ontario municipalities. J Assoc Off Anal Chem, **71**(2): 410–414.

Wilson Committee (1969) Report by the Advisory Committee on Pesticides and Other Toxic Chemicals. Further review of certain persistent organochlorine pesticides used in Great Britain. London, Her Majesty's Stationery Office, pp 90–100.

Wilson JG & Earley JJ (1986) Pesticide and PCB levels in the eggs of shag *Phalacrocorax aristotelis* and cormorant *Phalacrocorax carbo* from Ireland. Environ Pollut (Ser B), **12**: 15–26.

Wit SL (1971) [Persistent insecticides in Dutch body fat.] Chem Weekbl, **67**(5): 11–14 (in Dutch).

Witherup S, Stemmer KL, Taylor P, & Bietsch P (1970) The Incidence of Neoplasms in Two Strains of Mice Sustained on Diets Containing Endrin. Unpublished report, Cincinnati, Ohio, Kettering Laboratory, submitted to WHO by Shell.

Wolfe HR, Durham WF, & Armstrong JF (1963) Health hazards of the pesticides endrin and dieldrin: hazards in some agricultural uses in the Pacific Northwest. Arch Environ Health, **6**: 458–464.

Wolfe HR, Durham WF, & Armstrong JF (1967) Exposure of workers to pesticides. Arch Environ Health, **14**: 622–633.

Wolman AA & Wilson AJ Jr (1970) Occurrence of pesticides in whales. Pestic Monit J, **4**(1): 8–10.

Wüthrich C, Müller F, Blaser O, & Marek B (1985) [Pesticides and other chemical residues in Swiss diet samples.] Mitt Geb Lebensmittel Hyg, **76**: 260–276 (in German with English summary).

Wuu KD & Grant WF (1966) Morphological and somatic chromosomal aberrations induced by pesticides in barley (*Hordeum vulgare*). Can J Genet Cytol, **8**: 481–501.

Wuu KD & Grant WF (1967a) Chromosomal aberrations induced by pesticides in meiotic cells of barley. Cytologia, **32**: 31–41.

Wuu KD & Grant WF (1967b) Chromosomal aberrations induced in somatic cells of *Vicia faba* by pesticides. Nucleus, **10**(1): 37–46.

Yakushiji T, Watanabe I, Kuwabara K, Yoshida S, Hori S, Fukushima S, Kashimoto T, Koyama K, & Kunita N (1979) Levels of organochlorine pesticides and polychlorinated biphenyls (PCBs) in mothers milk collected in Osaka prefecture from 1969-1976. Arch Environ Contam Toxicol, **8**: 59–66.

Yarbrough JD, Roush RT, Bonner JC, & Wise DA (1986) Monogenic inheritance of cyclodiene insecticide resistance in mosquitofish, *Gambusia affinis*. Experientia (Basel), **42**: 851–853.

Young RA & Mehendale HM (1986) Effect of endrin and endrin derivatives on hepatobiliary function and carbontetrachloride-induced hepatotoxicity in male and female rats. Food Chem Toxicol, **24**(8): 863–868.

Zabik MJ, Schuetz RD, Burton WL, & Pape BE (1971) Photochemistry of bioactive compounds. Studies of a major photolytic product of endrin. J Agric Food Chem, **19**(2): 308–313.

Zavon MR, Hine CH, & Parker KD (1965) Chlorinated hydrocarbon insecticides in human body fat in the United States. J Am Med Assoc, **193**(10): 181–183.

Zeiger E (1987) Carcinogenicity of mutagens: predictive capability of the *Salmonella* mutagenesis assay for rodent carcinogenicity. Cancer Res, **47**: 1287–1296.

Zeiger E, Anderson B, Haworth S, Lawlor T, Mortelmans K, & Speck W (1987) *Salmonella* mutagenicity tests: III. Results from the testing of 255 chemicals. Environ Mutagen, **9** (suppl9): 1–110.

Zimmerli B & Marek B (1973) [The pesticide load of the Swiss population.] Mitt Geb Lebensmittel Hyg,, **64**(4): 459–479 (in German with English summary).

ANNEX I

CHEMICAL NAMES OF ENDRIN AND ITS METABOLITES

Two main systems are currently used for the nomenclature of cyclodiene insecticides: 'polyhydroaromatic' names, used by Chemical Abstracts (American Chemical Society) and the International Union for Pure and Applied Chemistry (IUPAC), and the von Baeyer/IUPAC system for polycyclic aliphatic compounds. Benson (1969) and Bedford (1974) proposed that the latter system be used for the cyclodiene insecticides.

The 'polyaromatic' system has, unfortunately, been subject to historical variation, and there are differences between the IUPAC, British and American conventions for defining the three-dimensional stereochemistry in this system. As a consequence of differences in the numbering of carbon atoms in the two systems and the modification of the Chemical Abstracts 'polyaromatic' name for dieldrin since 1971, considerable confusion can arise in the nomenclature of metabolites. The possible misunderstandings that may occur, particularly among people who are not familiar with the various conventions of chemical nomenclature, are illustrated by the different names that are given to the major metabolite of endrin; this one compound may be designated as:

> *anti*-9-hydroxyendrin (former Chemical Abstracts system)
> *anti*-8-hydroxyendrin (current Chemical Abstracts system)
> *anti*-12-hydroxyendrin (von Baeyer/IUPAC system).

A useful discussion of nomenclature was given by Brooks (1974).

The chemical names for endrin and its metabolites are summarized in Table 30.

Table 30. Chemical nomenclature of endrin and its metobolites

Trivial names[a]	Polycyclic aliphatic name (von Baeyer/ IUPAC)	Alternative or former names
Endrin (I)	1,8,9,10,11,11-Hexachloro-4,5-*exo*-epoxy-2,3-7, 6-*endo*-2,1-7,8-*endo*-tetracyclo[6.2.1.1^{3,6}.0^{2,7}]-dodec-9-ene	1,2,3,4,10,10-Hexachloro-6,7-epoxy-1,4, 4a,5,6,7,8,8a-octahydro-1,4-*endo*,*endo*-5,8-demethanonaphthalene (former CAS name) 1aa,2b,2ab,3a,6a,6b,7b,7a)-3,4,5,6,9,9-Hexachloro-1a,2,2a,3,6,6a,7,7a,-octahydro-2,7-3,6-dimethanonaphth[2,3-b]oxirene (current CAS name) (IR,4S,4aS,5S,7R,8R,8aR)-1,2,3,4,10,10-Hexachloro-1,4,4a,5,6,7,8,8a-octahydro-6,7-epoxy-1,5:5,8-dimethanonaphthalene (current IUPAC name)
syn-12-Hydroxyendrin (II) (9-*syn*-hydroxyendrin)	1,8,9,11,11-Hexachloro-4,5-*exo*-epoxy-12-(*syn*-epoxy)hydroxy-2,3-7,6-*endo*-2,1-7,8-*endo*-tetracyclo[6.2.1.1^{3,6}.0^{2,7}] dodec-9-ene	
anti-12-Hydroxyendrin (III) (9-*anti*-hydroxyendrin)	1,8,9,10,11,11-Hexachloro-4,5-*exo*-epoxy-12-(*anti*-epoxy)hydroxy-2,3-7,6-*endo*-2,1-7,8-*endo*-tetracyclo[6.2.1.1^{3,6}.0^{2,7}]dodec-9-ene	
3-Hydroxyendrin (IV) (5-hydroxyendrin)	1,8,9,10,11,11-Hexachloro-4,5-*exo*-epoxy-3-hydroxy-2,3-7,6-*endo*-2,1-7,8-*endo*-tetracyclo-[6.2.1.1^{3,6}.0^{2,7}] dodec-9-ene	

Annex I

Table 30. (contd)

Trivial names[a]	Polycyclic aliphatic name (von Baeyer/ IUPAC)	Alternative or former names
12-Ketoendrin (V) (9-ketoendrin)	1,8,9,10,11,11-Hexachloro-4,5-*exo*-epoxy-2,3-7,6-*endo*-2,1-7,8-*endo*-tetracyclo[6.2.1.1^{3,6}.0^{2,7}]-dodec-12-one	
Endrin *trans*-diol (IV)	1,8,9,10,11,11-Hexachloro-4,5-(*exo*)*trans*-dihydroxy-2,3-7,6-*endo*-2,1-7,8-*endo*-tetracyclo[6.2.1.1^{3,6}.0^{2,7}] dodec-9-ene	

[a]Roman numerals in parentheses refer to the structures in Figure 2.

ANNEX II

MEDICAL TREATMENT OF ENDRIN POISONING

1. ## Symptoms of poisoning

Endrin is readily absorbed and is toxic when taken by mouth, by skin contact (especially liquid formulations), and by inhalation. It stimulates the central nervous system, and an oral dose of 0.25 mg/kg body weight can cause convulsions in humans. Following accidental ingestion or gross over-exposure, symptoms appear between 20 min and 12 h and may include headache, dizziness, nausea, vomiting, weakness in the legs, and convulsions, sometimes leading to death.

Organochlorine compounds can cause respiratory depression, and they may sensitize the heart to endogenous catecholamines, leading to ventricular fibrillation and cardiac arrest in severe cases. Respiratory depression may lead to metabolic acidosis, and if necessary blood gases should be checked. Use of an electrocardiographic monitor is recommended if symptoms are severe.

Endrin is eliminated very quickly from the blood and can be detected for only 1 or 2 days even after massive over-exposures. Signs and symptoms of poisoning occur only at levels in whole blood of above 0.05 µg/ml.

2. ## Medical treatment

Medical treatment is largely symptomatic and supportive and is directed against convulsions and hypoxia. If endrin is swallowed, the stomach should be emptied as soon as possible by careful gastric lavage (with a cuffed endotracheal tube already in place), avoiding aspiration into the lungs. In a rural situation where this is not feasible, vomiting should be induced immediately. This should be followed by (intragastric) administration of 50 g of activated charcoal and 30 g of magnesium or sodium sulfate in a 30% aqueous solution. Oily purgatives are contraindicated, and no fats, oils, or milk should be given.

Annex II

If convulsions occur, anticonvulsants should be given immediately but slowly, and repeated as necessary. Diazepam can be given at 10 mg (children, 1–5 mg) intravenously; thiopental sodium or hexobarbital sodium can be given intravenously at a dose of 10 mg/kg, with a maximum total dose of up to 750 mg for an adult; or paraldehyde can be given at 5 ml by intramuscular injection. These short-acting anticonvulsants should always be followed by phenobarbital given orally at 3 mg/kg (up to 200 mg for an adult), or phenobarbital sodium given intramuscularly at 3 mg/kg (up to 200 mg for an adult).

Morphine and its derivatives, adrenaline and noradrenaline, should never be given.

The airway must be kept unobstructed. Respiratory inadequacy, which may be accentuated by barbiturate anticonvulsants, should be corrected, and oxygen and/or artificial ventilation may be needed.

A guideline for the management of major status epilepticus is added as Annex III.

ANNEX III

MANAGEMENT OF MAJOR STATUS EPILEPTICUS IN ADULTS[a]

1. Initial management

1. Assess the patient, verify the diagnosis, remove false teeth, place the patient in a lateral semi-prone position, and establish an airway.

2. Give diazepam intravenously (see Note 1, below), usually at 10 mg in 2 ml (0.15–0.25 mg/kg), followed immediately by a further 10 mg (2 ml) over 1–2 min. This may be repeated according to response.

3. Take blood to measure levels of anticonvulsant drug, ethanol, and blood sugar (5 ml of blood in a sugar tube); a sample to measure calcium (5 ml in a plain tube); and a drop of blood to determine blood glucose.

4. If the latter measurement shows low blood glucose level, 25 ml of 50% glucose should be given intravenously, preferably by catheter and not into a small distal vein. If ethanol is likely to be present, give thiamine intravenously at 100 mg.

5. Give phenytoin intravenously at 250 mg in 5 ml (10–15 mg/kg) no faster than 50 mg (1 ml)/min by infusion pump or slow intravenous injection (see Note 2, below).

2. If fits continue, transfer patient to the intensive care unit and consult an anaesthetist

6. Give chlormethiazole intravenously at 8 mg/ml: a loading dose of up to 800 mg (100 ml) over 10 min at 10 ml/min, maintained with 0.5–1 ml/min (4–8 mg).

---

[a] Adapted from guidelines issued at Guy's Hospital, London

Annex III

7. Give thiopentone intravenously at 5 mg/kg as a loading dose, then 1–3 mg/kg per h to a maximum blood level of 100 mg/litre.

8. If this fails, consult a neurologist.

3. Notes

1. Diazepam: A bolus injection of 10 mg may cause respiratory depression and hypotension, which may be pronounced if there is concurrent use of other central nervous system depressant drugs, especially phenobarbital.

   Diazepam must *not* be given intramuscularly:
   —added to an intravenous infusion
   —with phenobarbital, unless artificial ventilation is available.

   Rectal administration of diazepam (using a rectal administration set), at 5 or 10 mg in 2.5 ml, may be used for the immediate treatment of epilepsy instead of intravenous diazepam.

2. Phenytoin must *not* be given:
   —intramuscularly
   —by central line
   —into a dextrose infusion
   —with any other drug.

   Intravenously administered phenytoin should be monitored by continuous electrocardiographic recording. If this is not available, it may be safer to use a diluted solution of 250 mg (5 ml) in 250 ml of normal saline, no faster than 50 mg/min. The diluted solution should be used immediately provided there is no evidence of precipitation (this use of phenytoin is not licensed).

4. Options

The following drugs may also be used:

1. Paraldehyde: 2 x 5 ml by separate deep intramuscular injection or 10 ml diluted in 100 ml of normal saline given intravenously over 10–15 min. Note: Paraldehyde should be administered only with glass syringes.

2. Phenobarbital: 200 mg/ml, should not be given intravenously except when artificial ventilation is available, and not at all if the patient normally takes phenobarbital. The maximal rate of infusion is 100 mg/min to a maximum dose of 15 mg/kg.

3. Lignocaine: 100 mg by slow intravenous injection, followed by 50–100 mg in 250 ml of 5% dextrose at 1–2 mg/min. Note: This treatment must be monitored by electrocardigram.

4. Diazepam: 10 mg in 2 ml intravenously, or 40 mg in 500 ml of 5% dextrose at a maximal infusion rate of 100 mg/h.

5. Sodium valproate: 400 mg in 4 ml, or 400-800 mg intravenously over 3–5 min (up to 10 mg/kg), followed by intravenous. infusion to a maximum of 2.5 g/day (unlicensed).

Paediatric doses

For children, dosing should be adapted as follows:

Diazepam:	0.2–0.3 mg/kg intravenously
Phenytoin:	10–20 mg/kg intravenously
Chlormethiazole:	5–10 mg/kg per h, equivalent to 0.6–1.25 ml/kg per h

RESUME ET EVALUATION; CONCLUSIONS; RECOMMANDATIONS

Résumé et évaluation

Exposition

L'endrine est un insecticide organochloré utilisé depuis les années 1950 contre toute sorte de ravageurs, qui s'attaquent notamment au coton mais également au riz, à la canne à sucre, au maïs et à d'autres cultures. On l'utilise également comme rodenticide et avicide. Il est disponible dans le commerce sous forme de poudres, de granulés, de pâtes et de concentrés émulsionnables.

L'endrine pénètre principalement dans l'atmosphère par volatilisation et dispersion. En général, la volatilisation se produit après épandage sur le sol et sur les récoltes et elle est tributaire de nombreux facteurs comme la teneur en matières organiques et en eau du sol, l'humidité, les courants aériens et l'aire foliaire des végétaux.

C'est principalement par lessivage à partir du sol que se produit la contamination des eaux superficielles. Les précipitations, qu'il s'agisse de neige ou de pluie, n'ont qu'une part négligeable dans cette contamination.

Localement, une contamination peut également se produire par suite du déversement d'effluents industriels ou de négligences dans les techniques d'épandage.

C'est principalement par suite d'un épandage direct sur les terrains et les récoltes que l'endrine pénètre dans le sol. Elle peut y être retenue, transportée ou dégradée, en fonction d'un certain nombre de facteurs. C'est dans les sols riches en matières organiques que la rétention est la plus importante. La persistance de l'endrine dépend dans une large mesure des conditions locales; sa demi-vie dans le sol peut aller jusqu'à 12 ans. La disparition de l'endrine présente en surface s'effectue principalement par volatilisation et photodécomposition. Sous l'influence de la lumière solaire (rayonnement ultra-violet), l'endrine est isomérisée en delta-cétoendrine. En présence de lumière solaire intense, on a observé une isomérisation de 50% de l'endrine en l'espace de sept jours. L'isomérisation peut également s'effectuer par action microbienne (champignons et bactéries), notamment en anaérobiose.

Les invertébrés aquatiques et les poissons absorbent rapidement l'endrine présente dans l'eau mais, transvasés dans une eau non contaminée, les poissons exposés éliminent sans délai le pesticide. En cas d'exposition continue, le facteur de bioconcentration peut atteindre 14–18 000.

Il est possible que les invertébrés terricoles absorbent facilement l'endrine. La présence occasionnelle de faibles quantités d'endrine dans l'air ainsi que dans les eaux de surface, notamment destinées à la consommation, en zone agricole, n'a guère d'importance au point de vue de la santé publique. La seule voie d'exposition importante est la voie alimentaire. En général, toutefois, les quantités ingérées se situent très largement en-dessous de la dose journalière admissible qui a été fixée à 0,0002 mg/kg de poids corporel en 1970 (FAO/OMS, 1971).

1.2 Absorption, métabolisme et excrétion

Contrairement à la dieldrine, son stéréoisomère, l'endrine est rapidement métabolisée par l'organisme animal et, comparativement à d'autres composés de structure chimique semblable, elle s'accumule très peu dans les tissus adipeux.

L'absorption et l'excrétion sont rapides après administration orale à des rats et la demi-vie biologique se situe entre 1 et 6 jours selon les quantités ingérées. Un régime stationnaire, c'est à dire un état d'équilibre entre la quantité excrétée et la dose ingérée, s'établit au bout de 6 jours. On constate une différence entre les deux sexes en ce sens que les mâles excrètent l'endrine et ses métabolites par la voie biliaire plus rapidement que les femelles, d'où une moindre accumulation de pesticides dans les tissus adipeux des mâles. Les rats excrètent ce composé principalement dans leurs matières fécales sous forme d'endrine, d'*anti*-12-hydroxyendrine ainsi que sous la forme d'un dérivé hydroxylé de l'endrine, en l'espace de 24 heures (70-75%); un troisième métabolite, la 12-cétoendrine, s'accumule dans les tissus. Les lapins excrètent 50% des métabolites de l'endrine par la voie urinaire, l'excrétion urinaire n'étant que de 2% chez le rat; dans les matières fécales des lapins, on ne retrouve que de l'endrine non modifiée.

Des vaches à qui l'on avait administré de l'endrine à raison de 0,1 mg/kg de nourriture pendant 21 jours en ont excrété jusqu'à 65% sous forme de métabolites urinaires, 20% sous forme de métabolites fécaux ou d'endrine non modifiée et 3% dans leur lait, cette fois, principalement sous

Résumé

forme d'endrine non modifiée. Chez ces vaches, les résidus atteignaient 0,003–0,006 mg/litre dans le lait, 0,001–0,002 mg/kg dans la viande, et 0,02–0,1 mg/kg dans la graisse.

Chez des poules pondeuses ayant reçu une alimentation additionnée d'endrine, on a observé des résidus (selon la dose ingérée) qui atteignaient 0,1 mg/kg dans la chair, 1 mg/kg dans la graisse, 0,2–0,3 mg/kg dans les œufs (jaune), 0,2 mg/kg dans les reins et 0,5 mg/kg dans le foie. Sauf dans le cas du foie et des reins, les résidus présents étaient essentiellement formés d'endrine non modifiée. Environ 50% de la quantité d'endrine administrée a été excrétée dans les matières fécales, principalement sous la forme de métabolites.

Chez l'homme, le rat, le lapin, la vache et la poule, le principal métabolite de l'endrine est l'*anti*-12-hydroxyendrine, accompagnée de ses sulfo- et glucuro-conjugués. On trouve également 4 autres métabolites, mais en quantités minimes. Dans les tissus et le lait on retrouve essentiellement de l'endrine non modifiée. Après épandage sur des végétaux, on a retrouvé de l'endrine sous forme non modifiée ainsi que deux produits de transformation hydrophiles.

1.3 Effets sur les êtres vivants dans leur milieu naturel

L'endrine n'exerce que des effets minimes sur les bactéries et les champignons terricoles. Aux doses de 10–1000 mg/kg de terre, le composé n'a aucun effet sur la décomposition des matières organiques, sur la dénitrification ou sur la production de méthane. L'endrine est très toxique pour les poissons, les invertébrés aquatiques et le phytoplancton; la CL_{50} à 96 h, est dans la plupart des cas inférieure à 1,0 µg/litre. La dose nocive la plus faible observée au cours d'un test portant sur le cycle évolutif d'un crevette, *Mysidopsis bahia*, était de 30 ng/litre.

Les épreuves de toxicité aiguë effectuées sur des organismes aquatiques ont été pratiquées dans des aquariums ne comportant pas de sédiments; on peut penser que la présence de sédiments atténue l'effet de l'endrine. D'ailleurs la présence de sédiments fortement contaminés n'a guère eu d'effet sur les espèces de pleine eau, ce qui incite à penser que l'endrine fixée aux sédiments présente une faible biodisponibilité. On n'a pas pratiqué d'épreuves sur des animaux aquatiques vivant dans les sédiments.

Pour les mammifères terrestres et les oiseaux, la DL_{50} est de l'ordre de 1,0–10,0 mg/kg de poids corporel. Des canards de l'espèce *Anas platyrhynchos* qui avaient reçu pendant 12 semaines de l'endrine dans leur nourriture à des doses allant jusqu'à 3,0 mg/kg de poids corporel, n'ont présenté aucun effet délétère que ce soit sur la ponte, la fécondité ou l'éclosion des œufs.

Il semblerait que certaines espèces d'invertébrés aquatiques, de poissons et de petits mammifères résistent à l'action toxique de l'endrine; d'ailleurs l'exposition à divers pesticides organochlorés a pu entraîner la sélection de souches résistantes à l'endrine.

Dans des zones où existent des décharges industrielles et où l'endrine peut être entraînée par ruissellement à partir des champs traités, on a observé une mortalité parmi les poissons; par ailleurs, le déclin des populations de pélicans bruns (en Louisiane) et de caugeks (aux Pays-Bas) a été attribuée à une exposition à l'endrine et à d'autres dérivés halogénés.

1.4 Effets sur les animaux d'expérience et sur les systèmes *in vitro*

L'endrine est un pesticide fortement toxique dont les signes d'intoxication sont de type neurologiques. Chez les animaux de laboratoire, la DL_{50} par voie orale de l'endrine de qualité technique se situe dans les imites de 3–43 mg/kg de poids corporel; la DL_{50} dermique va de 5–20 mg/kg de poids corporel pour le rat. Il n'y a pas de différence notable concernant la toxicité aiguë par voie orale et percutanée entre le produit technique et les diverses formulations (concentrés émulsionnables ou poudres mouillables).

Des épreuves de courte durée portant sur la toxicité par voie orale de l'endrine ont été effectuées sur des souris, des rats, des lapins, des chiens et autres animaux domestiques. Chez les souris et les rats, les doses maximales tolérées ont été respectivement de 5 et 15 mg/kg de nourriture pendant 6 semaines (soit l'équivalent de 0,7 mg/kg de poids corporel). Les rats ont survécus à une dose de 1 mg/kg de nourriture pendant 16 semaines (soit l'equivalent de 0,05 mg/kg de poids corporel); les lapins sont morts après avoir reçu à plusieurs reprises une dose de 1 mg/kg de poids corporel. chez le chien, une dose de 1 mg/kg de nourriture (soit approximativement 0,025 mg/kg de poids corporel) administrée sur une période de 2 ans, n'a produit aucun effet.

Résumé

Du point de vue neurologique, les signes d'intoxication observés sont dus à l'inhibition de la fonction de l'acide gamma-aminobutyrique (GABA) à faible dose. Comme les autres hydrocarbures chlorés insecticides, l'endrine agit également au niveau du foie et la stimulation des systèmes enzymatiques intervenant dans le métabolisme des autres substances chimiques se manifeste, notamment chez la souris, par une diminution de la durée du sommeil induit par l'hexobarbital.

Des doses de 75–150 mg/kg appliquées sur l'épiderme des lapins sous forme de poudre sèche, tous les jours pendant deux heures ont entraîné des convulsions et la mort chez ces animaux sans toutefois provoquer d'irritation cutanée. Cette intoxication par voie générale sans irritation locale mérite d'être signalée.

Des études de toxicité et de cancérogénicité à long terme ont été effectuées sur des souris et des rats. Aucun effet cancérogène n'a été observé mais ces études présentaient un certain nombre d'insuffisances notamment la faible survie des animaux. Lors d'une étude de deux ans sur des rats traités par de l'endrine administrée dans leur nourriture, on a estimé à 1 mg/kg de nourriture, soit l'équivalent d'environ 0,05 mg/kg de poids corporel, la dose sans effets toxiques observables. Après administration d'endrine avec des quantité infinitésimales de substances chimiques cancérogènes pour l'animal, il n'a pas été possible de mettre en évidence d'effet tumoro-promoteur. Le Groupe de travail en a conclu que les données sont insuffisantes pour permettre de considérer l'endrine comme cancérogène pour l'homme.

Plusieurs études ont également révélé que l'endrine n'était pas génotoxique.

Dans la plupart des études, l'endrine s'est révélée non tératogène pour la souris, le rat ou le hamster, même à des doses toxiques pour la mère ou le fœtus. La dose sans effet nocif observable a été évaluée à 0,5 mg/kg de poids corporel chez la souris et le rat et à 0,75 mg/kg de poids corporel chez les hamsters. L'endrine n'a pas eu d'effets sur la reproduction des rats suivis pendant trois générations qui en recevaient dans leur nourriture à raison de 2 mg/kg (soit environ 0,1 mg/kg de poids corporel).

Un certain nombre de métabolites de l'endrine sont plus ou moins toxiques que le composé initial. Ainsi la delta-cétoendrine est moins toxique de l'endrine, en revanche la 12-cétoendrine est considérée comme le métabolite le plus toxique de l'endrine pour les mammifères, avec une DL_{50} par voie orale de 0,8–1,1 mg/kg de poids corporel chez le rat.

1.5 Effets sur l'homme

Plusieurs cas d'intoxication mortels ou non mortels consécutifs à un accident ou à une tentative de suicide ont été observés. Les cas d'intoxication aiguë non mortels résultant d'une surexposition accidentelle ont été observés chez les ouvriers d'une usine de production d'endrine. On estime que par voie orale, la dose mortelle est d'environ 10 mg/kg de poids corporel, une dose unique prise par voie orale de 0,25–1,0 mg/kg de poids corporel peut provoquer des convulsions.

C'est au niveau du système nerveux central que l'endrine exerce principalement son action. Après exposition à dose toxique, des signes d'intoxication peuvent faire leur apparition et se manifestent sous la forme d'un hyperexcitabilité et de convulsions, la mort pouvant survenir dans les 2–12 heures suivant l'exposition si un traitement approprié n'est pas institué immédiatement. En revanche, après une intoxication non mortelle, la récupération est rapide et complète.

L'endrine ne s'accumule pas dans le corps humain de manière importante. Chez 232 travailleurs exposés de par leur profession, on n'a pas constaté d'effets indésirables à long terme (durée d'exposition 4–27 ans) lors des examens médicaux pratiqués (durée de l'observation 2–29 ans). Le seul effet observé, indirectement d'ailleurs, consistait en une stimulation réversible des enzymes pharmacométabolisantes.

Des analyses ont été pratiquées dans de nombreux pays sur un grand nombre d'échantillons de tissus adipeux, de sang et de lait maternel sans qu'il soit possible de mettre en évidence la présence d'endrine. Le Groupe de travail attribue l'absence d'endrine dans ces échantillons à la faible exposition de la population général à ce pesticide et à sa métabolisation rapide.

En revanche la présence d'endrine a été décelée dans le sang (à des concentrations atteignant 450 µg/litre) et dans les tissus adipeux (à la dose de 89,5 mg/kg) chez les personnes décédées d'une intoxication accidentelle. Dans les conditions normales, on n'a pas retrouvé d'endrine chez les travailleurs exposés. Le seuil d'apparition des symptômes d'intoxication

Résumé

est estimé à 50–100 µg/litre de sang. On pense que la demi-vie de l'endrine dans le sang est de l'ordre de 24 heures.

2. Conclusions

L'endrine est un insecticide qui présente une très forte toxicité aiguë. Il peut entraîner des intoxications graves en cas d'exposition excessive due à une manipulation négligente lors de sa production, de son utilisation ou par suite de la consommation d'aliments contaminés. L'exposition de la population générale est principalement due à la présence de résidus dans les denrées alimentaires; toutefois on estime que la quantité d'endrine ingérée est en général très inférieure à la dose journalière admissible fixée par le Comité FAO/OMS d'experts des résidus de pesticides. Il n'y a pas de danger pour la population générale qui résulterait d'une exposition de ce genre à l'endrine. Moyennant de bonnes méthodes de travail et le respect des mesure d'hygiène et de sécurité, l'endrine ne devrait pas constituer un danger pour les ouvriers exposés.

Il est évident que des rejets incontrôlés d'endrine lors de la production, de la formulation et de l'utilisation de ce pesticide peuvent créer des problèmes écologiques dus à sa forte toxicité. Il n'est pas possible d'être aussi catégorique en ce qui concerne les effets que peut avoir son utilisation en agriculture sur la faune et la flore, encore que l'entraînement par ruissellement du pesticide puisse constituer une menace pour les poissons et les oiseaux piscivores. Le déclin des populations de certaines espèces d'oiseaux a été attribué à la présence de résidus élevés de divers organochlorés dans les tissus des adultes et dans les œufs. On a procédé au dosage de l'endrine chez certaines de ces espèces; toutefois il est difficile de faire la part des différents organochlorés qui sont en cause.

3. Recommandations

1. L'endrine ne doit être utilisée qu'en cas de nécessité et seulement lorsqu'il n'existe pas d'autre produit moins toxique.

2. Afin de préserver la santé et le bien-être des travailleurs et de la population générale, on ne doit confier la manipulation et l'épandage qu'à des personnes bien encadrées et bien formées qui appliqueront

des mesures de sécurité convenables et épandront le produit conformément aux règles de bonne pratique en la matière.

3. Il convient de s'entourer de toute les précautions nécessaires lors de la production, de la formulation, de l'utilisation en agriculture et du rejet de l'endrine afin de contaminer le moins possible l'environnement et en particulier les eaux de surface.

4. Les personnes qui sont habituellement exposées à l'endrine doivent subir des examens médicaux périodiques.

5. Il faut poursuivre l'étude épidémiologique des travailleurs exposés.

6. Dans les pays où l'on utilise encore de l'endrine, on devra contrôler la présence de résidus d'endrine dans les denrées alimentaires.

7. Au cas où l'on continuerait à utiliser de l'endrine, il faudrait obtenir davantage de données sur la présence, la destinée ultime et la toxicité de la 12-cétoendrine et de la delta-cétoendrine.

RESUMEN Y EVALUACION; CONCLUSIONES; RECOMENDACIONES

1. Resumen y evaluación

1.1 Exposición

La endrina es un insecticida organoclorado que se utiliza desde los años cincuenta para combatir muy diversas plagas agrícolas, sobre todo en el algodón aunque también en el arroz, la caña de azúcar, el maíz y otros cultivos. Se utiliza asimismo como rodenticida. En el comercio se encuentra en forma de polvos, gránulos, pastas y concentrado emulsionable.

La endrina se incorpora al aire principalmente por volatilización y arrastre aéreo. En general, la volatilización tiene lugar después de aplicarla a suelos y cultivos y depende de muchos factores, como el contenido de materia orgánica y agua del suelo, la humedad, el flujo de aire y la superficie cultivada.

La vía más importante de contaminación de las aguas de superficie es la escorrentía desde el suelo. La contaminación por precipitación en forma de nieve o lluvia es insignificante. Puede producirse contaminación local del medio debida a efluentes industriales y prácticas de aplicación poco meticulosas.

La principal fuente de endrina en el suelo es la aplicación directa a éste y a los cultivos. Puede quedar retenida, ser transportada o degradarse en el suelo, atendiendo a diversos factores. La retención más intensa se produce en suelos con contenido elevado de materia orgánica. La persistencia de la endrina depende en gran medida de las condiciones locales; su semivida en el suelo puede llegar a los 12 años. La volatilización y la fotodescomposición son los principales factores de la desaparición de la endrina de las superficies del suelo. La luz del sol (luz ultravioleta) induce la formación del isómero delta-cetoendrina. En verano, bajo insolación intensa, se observó que alrededor del 50% de la endrina se isomerizaba a esta cetoendrina en un plazo de siete días. Se produce transformación microbiana (en hongos y bacterias), especialmente en condiciones anaerobias, originándose la misma sustancia.

Los invertebrados acuáticos y los peces absorben rápidamente la endrina a partir del agua, si bien los peces expuestos transferidos a agua no contaminada pierden el plaguicida rápidamente. Se han registrado factores de bioconcentración de 14–18 000 tras una exposición continua. Los invertebrados del suelo también absorben fácilmente el compuesto.

La presencia ocasional de niveles reducidos de endrina en el aire y en las aguas de superficie y de bebida en zonas agrícolas reviste escasa importancia desde el punto de vista de la salud pública. La única exposición que merece consideración es la ingesta en la dieta. En general, no obstante, los niveles comunicados de ingesta se encuentran muy por debajo de la ingesta diaria admisible de 0,0002 mg/kg de peso corporal, establecida en 1970 (FAO/OMS, 1971).

1.2 Absorción, metabolismo y excreción

A diferencia de la dieldrina, su estereoisómero, la endrina se metaboliza rápidamente en los animales, y se acumula en muy pequeña cantidad en las grasas en comparación con compuestos de estructura química análoga.

En la rata, tanto la absorción como la excreción tras la administración oral se producen rápidamente; su semivida biológica es de 1–6 días, según la dosis administrada. Al cabo de 6 días se alcanza un estado de equilibrio en el que la cantidad excretada es igual a la ingesta diaria. Se observan diferencias de un sexo a otro: los machos excretan endrina y metabolitos con la bilis mucho más deprisa que las hembras, lo que produce una acumulación menor en el tejido adiposo de aquéllos. Las ratas excretan este compuesto principalmente en las heces en forma de endrina,*anti*-12-hidroxiendrina, y un derivado hidroxilado durante las primeras horas (70–75%); un tercer metabolito, la 12-cetoendrina, se acumula enlos tejidos. El conejo excreta el 50% de los metabolitos del compuesto enla orina, mientras que en la rata sólo el 2% se excreta por esta vía; en lasheces del conejo sólo se detecta endrina sin alterar.

Las vacas a las que se administró endrina a razón de 0,1 mg/kg de la dieta durante 21 días excretaron hasta el 65% en forma de metabolitos en la orina, el 20% en las heces, parcialmente en forma de endrina no alterada, y el 3% en la leche, también principalmente en forma de endrina. Estas vacas presentaron niveles residuales de 0,003–0,006 mg/litro en la leche, 0,001–0,002 mg/kg en la carne, y 0,02–0,1 mg/kg en la grasa.

Resumen

En gallinas ponedoras a las que se administró endrina por vía oral se observaron niveles residuales (dependientes de la dosis administrada) de hasta 0,1 mg/kg en la carne, 1 mg/kg en la grasa, 0,2–0,3 mg/kg en los huevos (yema), 0,2 mg/kg en el riñón y 0,5 mg/kg en el hígado. Salvo en el hígado y el riñón, los residuos encontrados estaban formados principalmente por endrina no alterada. Alrededor del 50% de la endrina administrada se excretó en las heces, principalmente en forma de metabolitos.

En el ser humano, la rata, el conejo, la vaca y la gallina, el principal metabolito biotransformado de la endrina es la *anti*-12-hidroxiendrina, junto con su sulfato y su glucur nido conjugados. Se encontraron cuatro metabolitos más, si bien en cantidades muy reducidas. En los tejidos corporales y en la leche se encuentra sobre todo endrina inalterada. Tras la aplicación de este plaguicida a plantas, se identificaron endrina inalterada y dos productos de transformación hidrófilos.

1.3 Efectos en los organismos del medio ambiente

El efecto de la endrina en las bacterias y los hongos del suelo es mínimo. Con dosis de 10–1000 mg/kg de suelo no se observó efecto alguno en la descomposición de materia orgánica, la desnitrificación ni la generación de metano. La endrina es sumamente tóxica para los peces, los invertebrados acuáticos y el fitoplancton: los valores de la CL_{50} a las 96 horas se encuentran en su mayoría por debajo de 1,0 µg/litro. El nivel sin observación de efectos más bajo en un ensayo de ciclo biológico del crustáceo Mysidopsis bahia se fijó en 30 ng/litro.

Los ensayos comunicados sobre la toxicidad aguda de la endrina para los organismos acuáticos se llevaron a cabo en acuarios sin sedimentos; cabría esperar que la presencia de sedimentos atenuara el efecto del insecticida. Los sedimentos muy contaminados ejercieron escaso efecto en las especies de aguas libres, lo que indica que la endrina ligada a los sedimentos tiene una biodisponibilidad reducida. Aún no se han llevado a cabo ensayos en animales acuáticos que viven en los sedimentos.

La DL_{50} para mamíferos terrestres y aves oscila entre 1,0 y 10,0 mg/kg de peso corporal. Los patos silvestres a los que se administraron 3,0 mg/kg de peso corporal durante 12 semanas no mostraron efecto alguno en la producción de huevos, la fertilidad o la eclosión.

Ciertas especies de invertebrados acuáticos, peces y mamíferos de pequeño tama o son resistentes a la toxicidad de la endrina; la exposición a diversos plaguicidas organoclorados llevó a la selección de estirpes resistentes a la endrina.

Se observaron muertes masivas de peces en zonas de escorrentía agrícola y descargas industriales; el declive de las poblaciones de pelícanos pardos (en Luisiana, EE.UU.) y de golondrinas de mar (Thalasseus sandvicensis) en los Países Bajos se ha atribuido a la exposición a la endrina en combinación con otras sustancias químicas halogenadas.

1.4 Efectos en animales de experimentación *in vitro*

La endrina es un plaguicida sumamente tóxico; los signos de intoxicación son de carácter neurotóxico. La DL_{50} por vía oral de la endrina de calidad técnica en animales de laboratorio oscila entre 3 y 43 mg/kg de peso corporal; la DL_{50} por vía cutánea en la rata es de 5–20 mg/kg peso corporal. No se ha encontrado ninguna diferencia en la toxicidad aguda por vía oral o cutánea entre los productos de calidad técnica y los formulados (concentrado emulsionable y polvos humectables).

Se han llevado a cabo experimentos de breve duración para estudiar la toxicidad por vía oral en el ratón, la rata, el conejo, el perro y animales domésticos. En el ratón y la rata, las dosis máximas toleradas durante 6 semanas fueron 5 y 15 mg/kg de la dieta (equivalentes a 0,7 mg/kg de peso corporal), respectivamente. Las ratas sobrevivieron tras una exposición a 1 mg/kg de la dieta (equivalente a 0,05 mg/kg de peso corporal) durante 16 semanas; los conejos murieron tras recibir dosis repetidas de 1 mg/kg de peso corporal. En el perro, no se observó efecto alguno tras la administración de 1 mg/kg de la dieta (equivalente aproximadamente a 0,025 mg/kg de peso corporal) durante más de 2 años.

La base neuroógica de los signos de intoxicación observados es la inhibición de la función del ácido gamma-aminobutírico (GABA) con dosis reducidas. Al igual que otros insecticidas a base de hidrocarburos clorados, la endrina afecta también al hígado, y se observa claramente la estimulación de sistemas enzimáticos que participan en el metabolismo de otras sustancias químicas, como lo demuestra, por ejemplo, la menor duración del sueño por hexobarbital en el ratón.

Resumen

Con dosis de 75–150 mg/kg aplicadas por vía cutánea en forma de polvo seco durante 2 horas al día se produjeron convulsiones y la muerte en el conejo pero sin irritación cutánea. Esta toxicidad sistémica sin irritación en el lugar de contacto resulta muy notable.

Se han llevado a cabo en ratones y ratas estudios prolongados de toxicidad y carcinogenicidad. No se observó efecto carcinogénico, pero estos estudios tenían ciertos defectos, entre ellos la reducida supervivencia de los animales. El nivel sin observación de efectos en cuanto a la toxicidad en un estudio de dos años de duración en la rata fue de 1 mg/kg de la dieta (equivalente a unos 0,05 mg/kg de peso corporal). No se demostró ningún efecto de favorecimiento de tumores cuando se ensayó la endrina en combinación con cantidades submínimas de sustancias químicas de conocido efecto carcinogénico en los animales. El Grupo de Trabajo concluyó que los datos de que se dispone no bastan para indicar que la endrina supone un riesgo carcinogénico para el ser humano.

En varios estudios se observó que la endrina no es genotóxica.

En la mayoría de los estudios no resultó teratogénica para el ratón, la rata o el hámster, ni siquiera con dosis suficientes para provocar toxicidad materna o fetal. El nivel sin observación de efectos adversos fue de 0,5 mg/kg de peso corporal en ratones y ratas y de 0,75 mg/kg de peso corporal en el hámster. La endrina no indujo efecto alguno en la reproducción de ratas estudiadas durante tres generaciones cuando se administró a razón de 2 mg/kg de la dieta (unos 0,1 mg/kg de peso corporal).

Algunos metabolitos de la endrina tienen toxicidades agudas iguales o más altas que el compuesto originario. El producto de transformación, la delta-cetoendrina, es menos tóxico que la endrina, pero la 12-cetoendrina se considera el metabolito más tóxico en los mamíferos, con una DL_{50} por vía oral en la rata de 0,8–1,1 mg/kg de peso corporal.

1.5 Efectos en el ser humano

Se han producido varios episodios de intoxicación mortal y no mortal, tanto accidentales como suicidas. Los casos de intoxicación aguda no mortal debida a exposición excesiva accidental se observaron en trabajadores de una planta de fabricación de endrina. Se ha calculado que la dosis que por vía oral provoca la muerte es de aproximadamente 10 mg/kg de peso corporal; la dosis única por vía oral que provoca convulsiones se fijó en 0,25–1,0 mg/kg de peso corporal.

El lugar principal de acción de la endrina es el sistema nervioso central. La exposición del ser humano a una dosis tóxica puede producir al cabo de pocas horas signos y síntomas de intoxicación tales como excitabilidad y convulsiones; la muerte puede producirse en las 2–12 horas que siguen a la exposición si no se administra inmediatamente el tratamiento apropiado. La recuperación después de una intoxicación no mortal es rápida y completa.

La endrina no se acumula en el cuerpo humano en grado significativo. No se comunicaron efectos adversos a largo plazo en 232 trabajadores expuestos (duración de la exposición: 4–27 años) bajo supervisión médica (tiempo de observación: 4–29 años). El único efecto observado fueron pruebas indirectas de una estimulación reversible de las enzimas metabolizadoras de fármacos.

No se detectó endrina en prácticamente ninguna muestra de tejido adiposo, sangre y leche humana analizadas en numerosos países. El Grupo de Trabajo atribuyó la ausencia de endrina en las muestras humanas a la baja exposición de la población general a este plaguicida y a su rápido metabolismo.

La endrina se detectó en la sangre (con concentraciones de hasta 450 µg/litro) y en el tejido adiposo (en concentraciones de 89,5 mg/kg) en casos de envenenamiento accidental mortal. No se encontró endrina en los trabajadores en circunstancias normales. El nivel umbral de endrina en la sangre por debajo del cual no se produce ningún signo o síntoma de intoxicación se ha fijado en 50–100 µg/litro. La semivida de la endrina en la sangre puede ser del orden de 24 horas.

2. Conclusiones

La endrina es un insecticida con elevada toxicidad aguda. Puede provocar envenenamiento grave en casos de exposición excesiva provocada por un manejo poco meticuloso durante su fabricación y uso o por el consumo de alimentos contaminados. El público está expuesto a la endrina principalmente por sus residuos en los alimentos; no obstante, los niveles de ingesta de endrina que se han comunicado están por lo general muy por

Resumen

debajo de la ingesta diaria admisible establecida por la FAO/OMS. Esas exposiciones en principio no constituyen un riesgo para la salud de la población general. Cuando se aplican buenas prácticas de trabajo, medidas higiénicas y precauciones de seguridad, es poco probable que la endrina suponga un riesgo para los trabajadores expuestos.

Está claro que las descargas no controladas de endrina durante su manufactura, formulación y uso pueden originar graves problemas ambientales asociados a su elevada toxicidad. Los efectos del uso agrícola del insecticida en la fauna y la flora están menos claros, si bien los peces y las aves ictívoras están expuestos por la escorrentía a partir de las superficies. El declive de las poblaciones de algunas especies de aves se ha atribuido a la presencia de niveles elevados de residuos de diversos compuestos organoclorados en los tejidos de adultos y en los huevos. Se ha medido la endrina presente en algunas de estas especies, pero es muy difícil separar los efectos de los distintos compuestos organoclorados presentes.

3. Recomendaciones

1. No debe utilizarse la endrina a menos que sea indispensable y sólo cuando no se disponga de una alternativa menos tóxica.

2. Para la salud y el bienestar de los trabajadores y de la población general, el manejo y el uso de la endrina se confiarán sólo a operarios bien supervisados y adiestrados que apliquen las medidas de seguridad adecuadas y utilicen la endrina de acuerdo con las prácticas agrícolas correctas.

3. La fabricación, la formulación, el uso agrícola y la evacuación de endrina se tratarán cuidadosamente para reducir al mínimo la contaminación del medio, en particular de las aguas de superficie.

4. Las personas expuestas regularmente a la endrina deben someterse a revisiones médicas periódicas.

5. Proseguirán los estudios epidemiológicos sobre las poblaciones de trabajadores expuestos.

6. En los países en los que aún se usa la endrina, deben vigilarse sus residuos en los alimentos.

7. Si sigue utilizándose la endrina, debe obtenerse más información sobre la presencia, el destino último y la toxicidad de la 12-cetoendrina y la delta-cetoendrina.

www.ingramcontent.com/pod-product-compliance
Ingram Content Group UK Ltd.
Pitfield, Milton Keynes, MK11 3LW, UK
UKHW021313180426
11947UKWH00015B/1211